CHILDHOOD CANCER:

ONE FAMILY'S JOURNEY THROUGH THE STORM

by
Peggy Timm

Foreword by
Ladonna Czachowski

Jewell Jordan Publishing, Llc
Oklahoma

Copyright © 2026 Peggy Timm

All rights reserved. This book, or any portion thereof, may not be reproduced or used in any manner whatsoever without the express written permission of the Publisher, except for the use of brief quotations in a book review.

NO AI TRAINING: Without in any way limiting the author's and publisher's exclusive rights under copyright, any use of this book to "train" generative artificial intelligence (AI) technologies to generate text is expressly prohibited. The author reserves all rights to license uses of this work for generative AI training and development of machine learning language models.

For information, address Jewel Jordan Publishing LLC
1205 S Air Depot Blvd, Suite 153, Midwest City, OK 73110

Interior Design by Mazharul
Cover Design by Sunita
Photographs from the Author

Library of Congress Control Number has been applied for.

Paperback ISBN: 978-1-7360906-8-8
eBook ISBN: 978-1-7360906-9-5

First Edition: 2026

Printed in the United States of America

Over 42 years ago, I started my pediatric nursing career at the University of Iowa Hospitals & Clinics (UIHC). The unit was organized by age – I was working on the toddler unit, which included children between the ages of 1-5 years. We cared for all diagnoses for children that required admission to the hospital, but not long into the assignment, something guided me to the pediatric oncology population. To this day, I'm not sure what it was, but I took care of a few children with cancer, and I knew it was where I wanted to be. 42 years later, I still hear people comment about how depressing that must be, but I find it to be quite the opposite. Caring for children and families who are often facing the most difficult times of their lives can have many rewards as you assist them in navigating this journey.

Throughout my career, I have watched the overall survival rate for childhood cancer grow from approximately 60% to over 80% of all childhood cancer diagnoses. After 4½ years as a bedside nurse, I transitioned into management, but pediatric oncology has always been part of my span of control. I have managed inpatient units, outpatient clinics, and full hematology-oncology service lines in 3 separate institutions. The sophistication and treatment of various childhood cancers has grown immensely over the past 40+ years, but regardless of the growing success, each child's new diagnosis of cancer is a new experience/nightmare to the family, which is suddenly facing one of the most difficult times of their life.

This book describes the journey of a family that faced their worst nightmare with a diagnosis of neuroblastoma in their 20-month-old daughter. Alicia's mother describes her personal feelings, how she worried about everyone else, the things people say that are helpful, and some that are not helpful. I have heard so many families talk about some of the examples she shares. People really cannot understand what this experience is like if they have not lived it, and as she describes, families on similar journeys are often most helpful to families facing a new diagnosis of childhood cancer. "I know how you feel" is never the right thing to say when speaking with a family in this situation unless they have truly experienced it.

Alicia's illness was a difficult one to treat. She is fortunate to have survived and is now leading a normal, healthy life. The author's story is very real and could be very helpful to families and others who are supporting someone with a new diagnosis of childhood cancer. I have had the pleasure of knowing Alicia's family since she was diagnosed, when initially I was one of her inpatient nurses. Long term, I kept in touch with her family through clinic visits, and eventually through summer camp where I had the pleasure of serving as a counselor for several years, and eventually as part of the camp medical team.

For those facing the new diagnosis of childhood cancer, whether as a parent, a loved one, or someone who wishes to support the family, this book provides the raw feelings, experiences, fears, etc. Readers will benefit by understanding the experience in more detail, validating that their feelings are not unusual, and identifying what is helpful to parents and family members in similar situations.

Kaye Schmidt, MA RN, CPHON ® NEA-BC

Peggy Timm's account of her daughter's diagnosis of neuroblastoma is vivid and honest. Timm reveals in piercing detail the resulting ongoing trauma for all involved. A must read to understand the turbulent ordeal of cancer survivors and their loved ones' endurance.

Jacinta Hart Kehoe, author of Mountain Lion Rises:
A Memoir of Healing

DEDICATION

To my family, Dick, Tony, Andy, Alicia. To all the children and their families who have had to battle through this STORM. Dark days during these struggles provide morning dawns that light the way for another day. To all the Warriors and Heroes! Continue to fight. To all the hematology/oncology doctors and hardcore nurses that care for these precious children every day, bless your hearts. Blessings to our family and friends for their support.

AND to my anchor in the storm, Ladonna.

Continue the WAVE at The University of Iowa
Stead Family Hospital!

CONTENTS

Dedication 7
Foreword. 9
    I. Diagnosis Day. 13
    II. Learning the Ropes 36
    III. Hospital Life. 49
    IV. The New Normal 66
    V. Realities & Frustrations/Smiles & Frowns/The
        Good and the Bad. 71
    VI. Siblings. 94
    VII. Cost, Gossip and Small-Town Support 101
    VIII. A World of Unknowns 106
    IX. Family and Friends: The Realities of Support. 110
    X. After the Good News 116
Finishing Up My Thoughts. 127
Acknowledgment 129

FOREWORD

As I was about to walk into my 3-year-old son's-room at the University of Iowa Hospitals and Clinics, a sobbing, petite, elderly woman grabbed my arm and said, "I can't believe my 20-month-old granddaughter has cancer. I can't believe it. Kids don't get cancer." I wrapped my long arms around her and whispered softly, "Yes, I can," and we hugged and cried, locked in a tight embrace. The woman was Peggy Timm's mom, and this hug was the beginning of a 40-plus-year relationship that Peggy and I have cherished as we traveled various roads on this life journey.

Over the years, Peggy would mention from time to time that she was thinking of dusting off the journal she had kept while her daughter, Alicia, was sick and hoped to make it a book someday about Alicia's cancer diagnosis and the time spent in the hospital for chemotherapy and other necessary treatments. Peggy would say she just wanted others to know how that journey affected the Timm family and many others. She would talk about letting people know how much a very simple act of kindness meant. Signs of love and support, no matter how large or small, were so crucial in keeping her going when she felt abandoned and overwhelmed with loneliness. Peggy walked and sometimes crawled every mile of the journey she writes about. She didn't stop when Alicia's treatments were finished. For 10 years, Peggy would spend her summer vacation week cooking at a children's cancer camp in Iowa as a way of helping others and giving back. Peggy was not a chef; Peggy and her husband are just two incredibly caring people who find it uplifting when they help others. They set an example for kindness, caring and concern.

Recently, Peggy mentioned again about dusting off the journal and finishing her book. However, she also said, "But I'm not a writer, I'm just a mom." What an important statement, "I'm just a mom." Peggy is a mom who loves her children, a mom who had to go from an ordinary mom to a constant advocate for her daughter in the dizzying world of medicine. Just a mom who spent two years traveling the chemo journey, followed by a lifetime of medical challenges and ups and downs related to Alicia's cancer and the painful treatment that followed. Just a mom who dealt with the loneliness of missing her two young sons who were cared for by family and friends while she stood guard in Alicia's sterile, lonely room at the University of Iowa Hospitals and Clinics. Just a mom missing those simple tasks of taking your toddler to the grocery store without fear of exposure to germs that may threaten her life. She was just a mom who missed her family of five being together. She was just a mom who worried about the medical expenses piling up. She was just a mom needing to take time off from work to care for a very sick child. She was just a mom who deeply felt compassion for other moms going through a similar experience. She was just a mom missing some of the important activities and adventures of her two sons at home. She was just a mom concerned about how her sons were feeling with mom not being around for them every fourth week of the month. She was just a mom wondering if her daughter would live or die. She was just a mom wondering if her daughter would ever go to school. She was just a mom worrying about how she would ever be able to tell her sons that their sister died. She was just a wife wondering how she and her husband would survive all of this. "I'm just a mom" can't describe all the things a parent has to become when she has a child with a serious illness.

As I read Peggy's manuscript, I found myself back in the emotional turmoil of those years of treatment, and the sounds, smells and loneliness of hospitalization when with your child. I also remember those hugs. Those hugs Peggy and I shared as we cared for our sick children. Hugs when the tears of pain and disappointment were rampant. Hugs when the tears of

FOREWORD

one little ray of good news would lift that heavy mass of concern off your shoulders for a brief moment, and then reality would set back in. Hugs when you were lonely, even though surrounded by medical personnel. Hugs when no words could be found. "This road is a damn long one," to quote Peggy. You don't know where it is taking you. Roadblocks or a new direction on the road pop up at any moment. You don't know where or when it will end. You have no choice but to stay on this road.

My son Philip was diagnosed with rhabdomyosarcoma just 15 days after his third birthday. What we were told was going to be something very simple, putting a tube in his eardrum to drain some fluid, turned into a parent's worst nightmare, childhood cancer. How did a child make this easier for his mom to tolerate the three to five days of in-hospital chemo every 4 weeks, when he knew it meant two days of almost constant vomiting followed by several days of just feeling yucky? When it was time to return for our in-hospital days of treatment, Philip just took his blankie, stuffed toy, and off we went. He kept busy by listening to music of his choice, talking with me, telling silly jokes, and watching to see how many semi-trailer trucks we spotted on our roughly 80-mile drive to the University of Iowa Hospitals and Clinics. Even though life was a mess, I would remind myself to cherish that precious gift of time I still had with Philip and pray that Philip's pain would not be intolerable this hospital stay. Our fun on the drive to Iowa City also kept my mind occupied and not thinking about what was ahead. On the drive home, however, Philip usually slept, exhausted from his treatment. This time for me provided a release from the emotions that had built up during our hospital stay and a chance to pull myself together as I prepared to return to my family and the challenges of life at home.

Unfortunately, 843 days into our rhabdomyosarcoma journey, Philip lost his battle. I cannot describe how grief feels, because it changes depending on the moment. I do know grief is less painful with friends by your side. Peggy and I traveled my road of grief together and continue to support each other to this day in the happy times and the challenging times. While Peggy's daughter survived her childhood cancer, never a day goes by that there isn't a small bit of fear medical troubles will surface again. When my road ended with Philip's death, the love, support, and hugs from my dear friend were a constant reminder that I was not alone traveling the road of grief.

For those wanting to support parents dealing with their children's serious illness of any type, as you read Peggy's book, you will experience what that daily journey is like. You will also notice that any simple gesture of kindness or concern will send a message of love and support. So please do not hesitate to think, will this insignificant gesture be of any help? It will, and it may be that one gesture is needed at the exact moment to give support to a family experiencing undesirable pain. For parents traveling this journey, try to always look for that one bright moment in each day, no matter how difficult it is, when you can hug your children or stroke their hands and tell your children you love them.

Hugs,
Ladonna Czachowski
Peggy's Friend

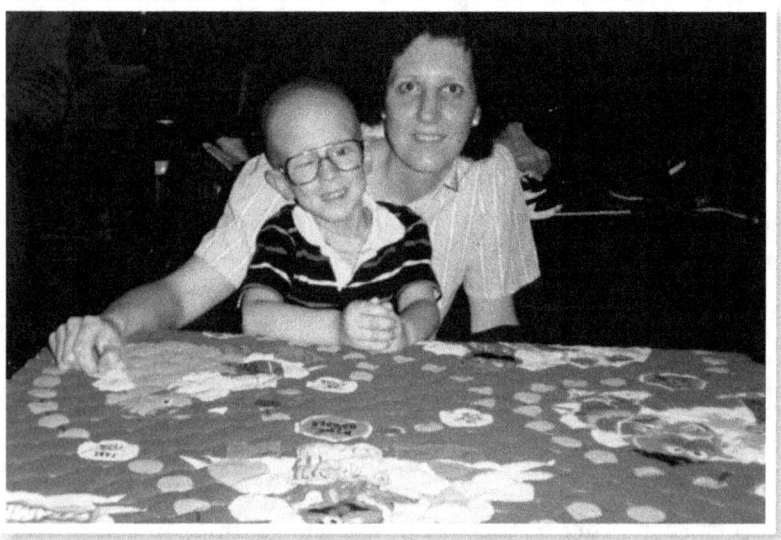

I
DIAGNOSIS DAY

Iowa weather in June is typically warm and humid, but the summer of 1983 seemed particularly warm, bordering on hot. Tipton, a small farming community with a population of approximately 3,000, in which I lived with my husband, Dick, our sons, Tony and Andy, and our daughter, Alicia, suffered from the same sweltering Iowa heat. Even today, those of us who live in small-town Tipton remain supportive of local businesses and one another. It is the county seat, and until 1994, Tipton was home to Cedar County's only stoplight. A second light was added in neighboring West Branch at the Herbert Hoover Presidential Memorial site.

Alicia was 20 months old and had been fighting a runny nose and cold for several weeks. I had taken her to the doctor in Tipton to see if we could get medicine to make her feel better. Dr. Chet Christiansen put her on penicillin, but when a week passed with no change, he put her on something stronger — and markedly more expensive — in hopes of getting the upper hand.

Just like the previous 70 or 80 years, on the last Sunday in June, we had our annual Lilienthal (my maiden name) family reunion at Tipton Park. Unfortunately, Alicia's cold hung on, and when combined with the heat and humidity, she wasn't at all herself. She had little energy and just wanted to be held. She wasn't the happy little girl we were accustomed to. So, in the middle of the picnic, I took her home for a nap. We would later return to the picnic.

I had been working in food service at The University of Iowa for 15 months. Since I always worked weekends, I had alternating Mondays and Thursdays off. The following Thursday, June 30th, I decided to take Alicia to her pediatrician in Iowa City for a well-baby care visit. I called the office and discovered that Alicia's regular pediatrician, Dr. Peter Wallace, was on vacation. Nonetheless, we could see his colleague, Dr. Stanley Hackbarth. That was fine with me. So, in the middle of the afternoon, I dressed Alicia in sandals and a little red and white outfit that her Grandma Lilienthal made her, and we headed out on our 40-minute drive to Iowa City.

After examining Alicia, Dr. Hackbarth suggested we go to Mercy Hospital for a chest X-ray. He thought she might have pneumonia, which had already been partially treated by the medicine prescribed by the Tipton doctor. I felt bad for Alicia, thinking she was that sick and no one had figured it out. That was the extent of my concern. Away we went to Mercy Hospital for a chest X-ray.

After the X-ray was taken, we were directed to the waiting area at the Mercy Hospital X-ray department, which was filled with natural light from the large windows. It had a tile floor and a row of chairs against one wall. While we waited, Alicia toddled back and forth, up and down the hallway between the chairs, giggling at the sounds her little hands made when she patted the chair seats.

After reading Alicia's X-ray, Dr. Hackbarth suggested she be admitted to the hospital for further testing. At that point, I was somewhat more concerned about Alicia and the severity of her illness; however, what scared me the most was thinking about the cost of these tests, inpatient care, and contacting our insurance company so there would be no payment problems. I didn't know if we had to get approval or a second opinion before admission.

Alicia and I headed to Admissions in the main part of the hospital. Sitting in the reception area, I called our insurance company to report that the doctor wanted to admit Alicia to the hospital for further testing. All this time, I still thought Alicia had pneumonia. We didn't have overnight bags or any personal items with us, but we checked in, and I called Dick to let him know we would be there.

"What kind of tests are they going to run? Are they just keeping her for the night?" Dick asked.

"I don't really know," I responded. "Dr. Hackbarth said he thought Alicia should be admitted. Maybe her pneumonia is worse than he originally thought, and he wants her in the hospital for observation," I said. "I called the insurance company, and they said since Dr. Hackbarth recommended admission, we did not need a second opinion before admitting her."

By the time Dick got off work, Alicia had a room, and he stopped by to visit us. He didn't stay long because he needed to get home to our sons. Tony was 9 years old, and Andy was 5 years old.

Dr. Hackbarth stopped by to visit us at about 6:30 p.m. He explained they were placing us in isolation because they feared Alicia might have tuberculosis, necessitating some additional testing, including blood work and urinalysis. I was not overly concerned. Although I thought tuberculosis was a thing of the past — I hadn't heard of anyone having TB for years — I also thought there was probably a logical explanation. Once we had an accurate diagnosis and received the right medicine, we would soon be back on our way to our happy home in Tipton with our three children.

That evening, I stayed in the room with Alicia while we waited for the additional tests. We played with toys and read books. She was perfectly content, just wandering around the room, chattering.

One of the nurses came to get Alicia for blood work. I was asked to wait in her room. Although Alicia went to the nurse without hesitation, she looked back at me as if to say, "Aren't you coming, Mommy?"

"Mommy will wait for you here," the nurse assured Alicia as if she read her thoughts.

When they returned, the nurse told me, "She only cried a little, Mommy. She is a brave girl." She then explained why I could not go with them, saying, "We ask parents not to go to the treatment rooms because children expect their parents to protect them from being hurt, and in this case, that isn't possible. Although you are not in the procedure room, we bring her back to you to be comforted."

The nurse also let me know that they changed Alicia's diaper so they could test her urine.

"OK," I replied. "Are we through with the tests for this evening?"

The nurse said yes and told me Alicia's dinner would arrive soon. She offered to sit with Alicia while I went to the hospital cafeteria for dinner. I thanked her for thinking of me, but I opted to stay with Alicia.

Dinner arrived, and Alicia ate well. The evening passed quickly, and Alicia settled into her big bed with bars on either side. I sat in a recliner beside her and watched her sleep for some time. Although I wasn't overly concerned about the tests or results, the night was long and sleepless. First, the chair was not particularly comfortable; then, the strange surroundings, nurses coming in and out of the room, and thoughts of what the next day would bring were not conducive to sleep.

Dr. Hackbarth returned before 6:30 a.m. the next morning. I was sitting in the rocking chair, holding Alicia, who was wearing her hospital-issued pajamas and slippers. I was still wearing the same clothes from the day before. Dr. Hackbarth, gentle in nature, sat down on the windowsill next to us. He asked if we'd had a good night.

"Is someone coming to be with you today?" he asked.

"No," I told him. "Dick is working, and we'll be fine getting through testing. I really don't mind. I have the day off to be with Alicia, and Dick doesn't like hospitals."

Dr. Hackbarth persisted. "I really think it would be better if you had someone here with you today. It could be a very long day, and I think it would be best if you weren't sitting alone."

"Oh, no," I assured him. "I don't see any reason for someone to waste the day sitting in the hospital when this is certainly something I am capable of handling."

Dr. Hackbarth repositioned himself closer to the edge of the windowsill and stared solemnly at the floor. "I think you need to get in touch with your husband and have him here with you today," he said somberly.

I turned my head to look at Dr. Hackbarth, unable to see his face. And while I did not question Dr. Hackbarth about why he suggested Dick join me, the seriousness in his voice finally struck me. I agreed to call Dick and have him come to the hospital. I began to wonder how serious this could be.

As we sat there, Dr. Hackbarth began to fill in some of the details:

"We have the results from Alicia's blood work and urinalysis," he told me. "Alicia's white blood counts are high, and so are her dopamine levels. So, we are going to schedule her for a bone marrow test."

Having heard those words all too recently when my cousin Gary was diagnosed with leukemia, tears were already welling in my eyes. Finally, I asked, "We aren't looking for TB, are we?"

CHILDHOOD CANCER

There was only silence as Dr. Hackbarth continued looking down at the floor. A natural darkness seemed to take over the room, and a sense of helplessness took over my body.

"I'm afraid we are up against neuroblastoma," he said softly. Then he explained, "It is a childhood cancer that we generally don't find in children over five years of age." He told me they wanted to do a computerized tomography scan, or as it is commonly called, a CAT scan, which provides detailed pictures of your organs, bones and tissues, along with some additional tests. They would then consult with an oncology specialist at The UIHC Pediatric Clinic. However, he told me that neuroblastoma was his diagnosis even before the next round of tests. Alicia's dopamine levels were extremely elevated, and it appeared there was a tumor in her chest.

I was stunned; then the questions flew from my mouth:

"A tumor? How could there be a tumor? What is dopamine? What does that level tell us?"

Dr. Hackbarth did his best to explain medical terminology to me as someone who: a) didn't understand much of anything medical beyond Band-Aids®, temperatures, and baby measles; and b) had just heard there was a possibility her child had cancer. He carefully answered my question about dopamine, explaining it is a hormone-like substance that facilitates critical brain functions in normal quantities. As a chemical messenger, dopamine is similar to adrenaline. It affects brain processes that control movement, emotional response, and the ability to experience pleasure and pain. He said, "Dopamine is a neurotransmitter."

I'm not sure why I kept asking questions, because I didn't understand any of his explanations. All I knew at this point was that Alicia's dopamine levels were at least four times the normal level, and her little body was indicating there were problems she was fighting. In this case, Alicia's body was battling a tumor.

DIAGNOSIS DAY

I remember just sitting there, numb. I looked at my daughter with her big brown eyes and strawberry-blonde, shoulder-length hair, trying to comprehend what I had just been told. I couldn't think of other questions to ask. Dr. Hackbarth's words cut like sharp knives and whirled in a dusty cloud above my head, making absolutely no sense at all.

Dr. Hackbarth went on to explain the tests that would be conducted, and the bone marrow procedure Alicia would undergo. I'm sure he realized I didn't fully comprehend what he told me, so he indicated he would be back later to answer any questions. He told me again that I needed someone to be with me.

Dick also worked at The University of Iowa at Burge Dining Hall. He worked early mornings, so he had already been at work for a couple of hours. I knew I needed to call him to come to the hospital, but I had no idea how I would tell him that his little girl was so sick. Dick lost his dad to cancer when he was just 11 years old.

I recall being calm during the phone call. "Dick?" I asked when he answered the phone.

"Yeah, what's wrong?" he asked immediately.

"Dr. Hackbarth was here and thinks you need to come to the hospital. They are going to do some additional tests." I was crying, but I was still able to be clear. "They are scheduling Alicia for a CAT scan and a bone marrow test. Dr. Hackbarth is afraid Alicia has a tumor in her chest, and these tests will give them more definite answers."

There was silence. Dick was seemingly as stunned as I was when I heard those same words.

"Dick?" I asked.

"Yeah, I'm here," he said.

"Can you get off work and come to be with us?" I asked.

"I'll be right there."

Dick appeared more quickly than I thought humanly possible. He was, of course, very concerned, but he remained strong and kept telling me we would get through the tests, and then hopefully, something else would show up, and it wouldn't be as serious as a tumor. He tried to keep reassuring me by saying, "First, we have to know what we are up against before we can know how to proceed. We have to think positively for Alicia."

"I know," I snapped. "I am being as brave as I can!"

"I know," Dick replied calmly. He was sitting on the same windowsill where Dr. Hackbarth sat when he delivered his initial findings an hour earlier. I was still rocking Alicia in the chair. We leaned toward one another and hugged. Only God knew what was ahead of us.

All I could do was cry. I couldn't even imagine not having our little girl. She was so sweet and so innocent, and she was just a baby. I had problems early in my pregnancy carrying Alicia, and I had already miscarried twice. So, the thought of losing her was just incomprehensible. Someone — probably the hospital staff — contacted our minister, Pastor David Franker, because he was there before noon. No one in Tipton was aware of what was going on.

Alicia was sedated for the CAT scan. While I vaguely remember them starting an IV to administer the sedative to prepare her for the scan, I mainly recall holding her tight, and that we rocked, and I cried.

Eventually, someone from the nursing staff came to take Alicia for the tests. Pastor Franker thought we should sit in a waiting area and take a break from her room. It was early afternoon. After we moved to the

DIAGNOSIS DAY

waiting room, Pastor Franker headed to the cafeteria, insisting that we eat something.

Although Dick had trouble sitting in any one place and did as much pacing as sitting, he sat beside me while Pastor Franker went to get the food.

"What are you thinking?" Dick asked.

"I'm just scared. I can't imagine life without Alicia. How could someone so young be so sick?"

I leaned against Dick, and he hugged me. I thought he was as much a pillar of strength physically as he was trying to be emotionally. We sat in silence.

Eventually, Pastor Franker returned to the waiting area with hamburgers and fries. Despite his kind gesture, I couldn't eat. I wondered how the tests were progressing and if Alicia was in pain or might be awake and scared. The nurses, particularly a nurse named Jackie, tried to comfort us.

Jackie sat with us for a few minutes to give an update, assuring the testing would not be painful for Alicia. "You have a beautiful little girl, and she has done very well. She will likely be tired from the tests and the sedation when she returns to her room. This is normal for children."

Jackie went back to stay with Alicia while she awaited the next test, and once she was taken for the remaining tests, Jackie returned to where Dick and I were waiting. She sat next to me and patted my hand. "Alicia's a real trooper, Mom," she told me. "We will all help you get through whatever you are facing."

Jackie was a small, blonde woman with lots of energy and an obvious love of children. We were able to be with Alicia between a couple of tests, and while I held Alicia, Jackie assured us that the tests were going well. One more test, and we would be through for the day.

At about 6:30 that evening, in the longest 12 hours of my life, Dr. Hackbarth returned to Alicia's room with the test results. The grave expression on his thin, handsome face told me it was not good news. Dick was sitting in the rocking chair, holding Alicia. She was still sleepy from the sedation, but I knew he needed to keep her close. He had been rocking her for some time.

"Yes," Dr. Hackbarth began, "the test results confirmed neuroblastoma." He was quiet for a moment as if to let this very bad news sink in, and then he explained briefly that the tumor was behind her heart and that it was a large mass.

One of the nurses offered to take Alicia from Dick and hold her or play with her if she woke up while we tried to digest this diagnosis, but Dick couldn't let go of her. The nausea I was feeling earlier just seemed to intensify. We sat there. Numb. Stunned. Neither of us could think of what we needed to ask the doctor. Dick had a blanket wrapped around Alicia. She was groggy from the medicine but perfectly content.

Finally, I relayed to Dr. Hackbarth that Alicia had been seen for her well-baby care and had received her shots, and that I didn't understand how something like this could have happened. Dick asked how long the doctors thought the tumor had been there. Dr. Hackbarth said he didn't know, but thought she might have been born with it, and that it had just started to grow. He told us that we are all born with undeveloped nerve cells, which usually develop normally. However, Alicia had a cluster or mass that did not develop and ultimately turned malignant.

Dr. Hackbarth said he would refer us to the head of the pediatric oncology unit at The University of Iowa Hospitals and Clinics (UIHC), Dr. C. Thomas Kisker, but that we would have to go home and wait out the July 4th weekend. I asked why we couldn't do the treatment at Mercy since we knew him and our pediatrician, Dr. Peter Wallace, and were more comfortable there. Dr. Hackbarth responded that the best place for Alicia was at UIHC because of its advanced testing equipment and the expertise of the oncologists. If we stayed with Mercy Hospital, we would still have to consult with the pediatric oncologists at UIHC. Further, he said someone from his pediatric group would have to come to Mercy to administer her chemotherapy. Dr. Hackbarth said his group could not have someone leave the practice and come to the hospital for such visits, and again, the best oncologists and specialists in this field were at the UIHC. He was so convincing that being at UIHC was the best thing for Alicia that we knew we needed to make the move without reservation.

However, I was emphatic about staying and doing more testing or checking into the UIHC immediately if that is what Dr. Hackbarth thought needed to be done. I panicked at the thought of going home and sitting and waiting. I had convinced myself we needed to keep moving, as every passing minute was crucial. I didn't want to waste three days doing nothing! How could we just sit and wait? Wouldn't that give the tumor time to grow much more? Wouldn't it be better if we were admitted and got started doing something?!

Dr. Hackbarth assured me we needed to complete all necessary testing before starting any treatment. He told us we needed to know exactly what we were up against and give the oncologists time to prepare the best possible protocol (treatment) for Alicia. With neuroblastoma being a relatively new cancer with little available written information, decisions had to be made regarding the course of treatment available to Alicia. Although that made perfect sense, the thought of sitting and doing nothing drove me crazy. He suggested we go home the next morning, which was Saturday, enjoy the holiday the best we could, and take time to explain things as we knew them to our boys and our families. We would have a few days to prepare for admission to the UIHC on July 5th. He would make the necessary arrangements for us to see Dr. Kisker and consult with him about the test results. He explained the treatment would probably entail chemotherapy and possibly surgery. However, we needed to discuss all options with the hematology-oncology teams at the UIHC.

Dr. Hackbarth left to allow us time to digest and understand the information he had given us, assuring us he would return later. "No doubt, you will think of things you want to ask; we will do our best to answer your questions and address your concerns," he said.

"Thank you, Dr. Hackbarth," I said. "I'm sorry, I can't even think of anything to ask."

"I understand," he said. "This is all unfamiliar material and pretty overwhelming. Take your time and make a list of your questions. Sometimes putting it on paper is easier. I'll be back."

With that, he disappeared into the hallway. Dick and I just sat and looked at each other, then at Alicia, in silence. Absolute shock. Dick's dad had died of cancer. My sister Vonnie's husband, Loren Cole, had died at the young age of thirty-five just a few years earlier. My cousin was sick . . . how on earth could God let this happen to a baby? To say this was the beginning of my faith being tested is an understatement.

It was about 7:30 p.m., still on that dreadful Friday, and we finally started considering our options for getting Alicia and me home on Saturday morning since Dick had to work all day. I had driven into Iowa City for Alicia's appointment, but I was certain I shouldn't drive home with Alicia. Dick suggested we call my mom and dad to see if they would come and get us and our car home the next morning. The problem: If we called them, we would have to tell Alicia's Grandma and Grandpa the preliminary diagnosis, and I didn't, for the life of me, know how on earth to do that. Dick called and asked them to come to the hospital yet that evening. He didn't tell them how sick Alicia was, but they knew it was something serious.

That I made Dick call was probably their first clue, and that we wanted them to come to Iowa City yet that evening was a second indication. My parents called my sister Vicki Meyer, and she brought them to Iowa City. I'm so thankful they weren't driving. My parents, who lived in Durant, Iowa, a small town about 45 minutes east of Iowa City, were unfamiliar with the city, and I was afraid they would be upset.

Dick and I just sat with Alicia in her hospital room and waited. How could this happen to a child — to our child? Alicia was still very groggy from the CAT scan anesthetic. We took turns holding her and rocking her. She was comfortable and content, drifting in and out of sleep. I remember the room was dark. I don't remember not wanting the lights on, but I do remember sitting in dark silence and rocking our girl. It seemed time was standing still yet swirling around us. Sometimes I felt like I was standing on the outside of the glass, watching everything happening. It certainly was a feeling of having no control — complete helplessness. We just had to watch and wait.

Mom, Dad, and Vicki arrived, and after seeing us, I suspect they knew instantly what we had was not good news. We gave them a summary of the past 36 hours and then explained what little we understood.

"Dr. Hackbarth, the pediatric specialist, is certain that Alicia has neuroblastoma," I told them. "Neuroblastoma is a childhood cancer; a tumor is in her chest. Therefore, we are transferring to the UIHC for further tests, evaluation, and treatment.

My sister, Vonnie, arrived shortly after Vicki and the folks. I don't know who called her, probably Mom. We got her caught up on the news. They were all as shocked as we had been. They were looking at each other and us, trying to figure out what to say. More tears were shed, and hugs were shared. The next couple of hours were a blur. I really don't even remember the conversations. I just held Alicia, watching her every move.

For some reason, I remember we had a wonderful male nurse that night. He came across the intercom system, asking Alicia if she'd like a Popsicle. In her still semi-anesthetized state, she was trying to figure out where that voice was coming from. We chuckled as she repeatedly tried to figure it out. The nurse brought her a Popsicle and some apple juice. Those around me in the room were talking, but I can't remember any particular conversation.

At about 10:30 p.m., Dick decided he had better get back to Tipton to tell the boys. They were with Dick's mother, Grandma Timm, and knew nothing about what was going on. I got Alicia ready for bed. She settled in, exhausted from her day. We all walked down to the hospital entrance so Dick, Vicki, my folks, and Vonnie could start for home. We ran into Dr. Hackbarth, and after introductions, he asked if we had any more questions. We stood and talked with him for a little while, and then he promised he'd be back in the morning. Vicki was taking Mom and Dad back home to Durant. Dick was going to tell his mom and the boys. Vonnie offered to stay, but I was sure I was fine and didn't need anyone there. She'd lost her husband to cancer 5 years earlier, and I didn't think she should be at the hospital reliving their hospital time. Vonnie suggested several more times that she would stay, but I continued to assure her I would be fine. As she turned to walk out the door, though, I said, in an anxious, scared voice, "Are you sure you wouldn't mind staying?"

"Of course not," Vonnie replied and came back to hug me.

I didn't know what I expected her to do, but suddenly I didn't want to be there alone. We walked slowly back to Alicia's room. She asked me if I was scared, and I told her I was, but I wasn't exactly sure what I was afraid of. She just squeezed my hand. I told her I didn't think it was fair to ask her to stay with all she'd been through, but she assured me she was all right to stay and that she didn't want her little sister to be alone. She also promised we would get through this once we knew what we were up against.

Vonnie called her daughter Lynne, who was almost 15 years old, to tell her she was staying with us at the hospital. It was storming — raining and lightning. And then I began to feel guilty for wanting Vonnie to stay when Lynne was home alone. I could hear Vonnie telling Lynne that Alicia was sick and that she would have to be admitted to UIHC for additional tests and a yet-to-be-determined treatment. I have always wondered how that conversation affected Lynne and how she felt when the hurt from losing her father to cancer was still so raw.

Vonnie and I slept in chairs in Alicia's room. I remember Vonnie asking if there was anything I wanted to talk about, but at that point, I still couldn't even think. She reached over and squeezed my hand. We didn't sleep much. I'm very thankful she was there with me.

Dr. Hackbarth was back early Saturday morning as promised. He explained who we would see and the tests we could expect when we checked into UIHC the following Tuesday. I knew Dick would be there with us. I knew he would want to meet Dr. Kisker and hear firsthand what they had to say regarding his daughter's test results and care. We had an appointment with Dr. Kisker in the clinic, after which Alicia would be admitted to the Pediatric Oncology Unit. I knew I would stay at the hospital with Alicia. The thought of leaving her there alone never occurred to me. Dr. Hackbarth explained there would be another CAT scan to confirm the earlier results, as well as blood work, urinalysis, a nuclear medicine bone scan, and probably another bone marrow test. The thought of redoing all those tests seemed draining for all of us.

Mom and Dad arrived at the hospital before noon on Saturday to transport us home to Tipton. "Good morning, girls," said Mom. "Are you ready to go home?"

"Yep," I said. "It doesn't take long to pack if you don't have any clean clothes or belongings with you!"

We said our goodbyes to the Mercy Hospital staff, who had been so good to us. They wished us well. It was difficult leaving there. There was a sense of security in that they knew as much as we did.

The next few days were just a matter of going through the motions. Some visitors and conversations are crystal clear, while others are blurry. I remember wondering what had happened to the stuffy nose Alicia checked into Mercy Hospital with, because she didn't seem to have it when we returned home.

We had to make arrangements for the boys and organize their schedules. We had no idea how long we would be in the hospital or what else we might learn. Looking back now to a time when I didn't think I'd ever forget a detail, I can't remember if the boys went to stay with Grandma Timm or if one of our siblings took them home. It seems they went to Grandma's so they would be close to home when Dick could be at home with them. Grandma Timm lived about six blocks from us. They were also involved with summer activities at the park in Tipton, so we wanted them to be able to keep going to those. The boys were confused about how sick their sister was. At 9, Tony was old enough to understand better, and he knew we'd lost family and friends to cancer. Andy was old enough to know his little sister was sick but didn't comprehend how sick. We explained to them we would do more testing and that their dad would be home every night to let them know anything we had learned. There were so many things we didn't understand at this point that it was very difficult to explain to the boys. Tony wondered if his little sister would die, and although we tried being optimistic, we couldn't promise her death wasn't a possibility. We explained we would have to get through the next week or two, and then we hoped to know much more. We asked the boys to put Alicia and our entire family in their prayers. We knew we would need help.

I woke up tired Sunday morning. I hadn't slept much, so I wasn't functioning well. Dick had gone to work. For him, having to go to work may have been a positive thing. He was certainly trying to be the strong, brave father figure, but I knew Alicia's illness reminded him of the loss of his father, causing him to fear what was ahead. He hates hospitals; hates visiting anyone in the hospital, even if it isn't serious. He didn't particularly like visiting me in the hospital when I had the kids or the couple of times I'd had surgery. He has all too vivid memories of seeing his father in the ICU — the last time he saw him alive. I knew this was wearing on him much more than he wanted anyone to know; nonetheless, he remained the constant stabilizing factor.

I remember feeling scared and worn, selfish and guilty all at the same time. I was so afraid of what was ahead. I have shared with many newly diagnosed families that the waiting part is the worst. Dick was right. Once you know what you are up against, you gather the available information and start moving forward with educated decisions. But, at this point, we just didn't know, and I was scared. I felt worn out from trying to make sense of everything we had been told. I tried being strong and positive in front of the boys so they would remain positive and not worry. Not only was I worrying about Alicia and wondering if we'd be able to keep her, but also how this would affect Tony and Andy, how Dick would cope, and how it would affect our aging parents and our entire families. I remember wishing Dick would just break down and have a good cry with me. Other than the night of diagnosis in the hospital, he hadn't been able to do that.

The selfish part of me just didn't understand how this could happen and why God would choose my daughter. I didn't want her to have to go through something like this, and why, how, could she be as sick as they were saying? I wanted to keep my daughter. I wanted our near-perfect family to go back to the way it was just a few days earlier. And then, I began feeling guilty. What had I done or eaten while carrying Alicia that could have caused this mass? What had I done wrong during my pregnancy to make this happen to her? She was only 20 months old, and that wasn't enough time to eat and breathe things harmful to her, so what had I done? I questioned how I could be selfish when my husband and siblings had already suffered such deep losses. I wasn't any better than any of them. What made me think I was exempt from such tragedies?

My brother, Tom, and his wife, Sally, visited Sunday. They had suffered the loss of a daughter, Meagan, just a couple of years earlier, when she was stillborn. How could I ask God to let us keep Alicia when he had taken Meagan from them? When he had taken Loren from Vonnie and left her to raise young children without their father? When Dick's family had already suffered too many losses? But I did. I asked God to help our little girl fight this disease and for all of us to be granted the strength it would take to get her through it. Most of all, I asked God to protect her from any pain and if he knew what was ahead, to please just do what he needed to do, but not to let her suffer in any way.

Several neighbors stopped by to let us know they were thinking of us. No one had any idea what to say; I understand now there isn't anything anyone can say to make you feel better. We were just overwhelmed.

Monday was July 4th and like the rest of the weekend, we tried making things as normal as possible for the kids, but of course, there was always the unknown weighing on our minds. Since Dick had to work, we didn't have plans. I worked around the house, trying to make sure it was clean and in order. I started packing suitcases for Alicia and me. Not knowing how long we would be there, I packed a few days' worth of clothes and personal items and figured Dick could bring anything else we needed when he came to see us.

The boys wanted to go to the fireworks display at the park. I just couldn't bear the thought of all the people who were going to ask how Alicia was and expect to be told the treatment and prognosis. I agreed to have Dick drive the van down to the park, and we'd sit in the van and watch the fireworks, but I couldn't go sit where people would ask too many questions. I know most people are concerned, but some want to know so they have something to report at their next coffee gathering, and I didn't care to sort one from the other.

People should understand cancer is not contagious. Cancer is not something you catch at the store, the park, or at church. Some of our friends really stepped in, offering help and support. Some shied away, and it seemed hardest for our friends who had a child the same age as Alicia. Part of the problem is a lack of knowledge about the disease. Part may be just not knowing what to say. Alicia's condition was neither their fault nor contagious, and people need to understand there is no "right thing" to say. In retrospect, I'd also say people need to think before they speak.

A friend of the family approached me soon after Alicia's diagnosis, and being a mother and grandmother herself, I assumed she was going to offer empathy and concern.

"How is Alicia feeling?" she asked.

"Pretty well so far," I responded. "She seems to be tolerating the tests as well as anyone could expect."

"This could be a very long process for all of you," she indicated.

"Yeah, it likely will be," I said, being realistic.

"Maybe it would be better if you would lose her now before you become any more attached," she said.

I just looked at her. I hope the look on my face was answer enough, because no words would come out of my mouth.

How could anyone say such a thing? How could anyone become more or less attached to his or her child? To this day, I still haven't figured out the logic behind that statement.

We made it through the horribly long weekend, just waiting for Tuesday to arrive. Between Dick working the entire weekend and taking the boys to see the fireworks, we had little chance to discuss what lay ahead of us. We didn't have any idea what the future held, but Dick remained strong and encouraged us to think positively and wait for the test results. He wanted to know all the facts. Dick remained the calmer, more level-headed parent, while I was the more panicked, worried one.

It was finally Tuesday, and we were due at the hospital first thing that morning. It was extremely difficult leaving the boys behind. We shared long hugs, "I love you's," and some tears, but I'm sure it was all the unknowns — the fear — that everyone was feeling. We assured the boys that their dad would be back as soon as he could to tell them anything we had learned. My Mom and Dad picked Dick, Alicia, and me up and took us to the hospital. I felt so sorry for them. Grandparents not only worry about the grandchild who is ill, but also their child who is suffering. I think, as parents, we just kept plugging along and trying to move forward with the sick child and the other children at home, while grandparents had more time to worry ... about everyone and everything. This was an extremely difficult time for both my parents and Dick's Mom. I learned very early on in this experience that being in a supportive role is never easy. Parents, siblings, grandparents, aunts, uncles, cousins, and close friends all have fears. Everyone handles these issues differently, and the relationship to the sick child certainly factors into the ability to cope. I have been so very thankful we lived close to family and could rely on all of them.

As we pulled into the parking ramp at the UIHC, I remember this overwhelmingly sick feeling. The buildings looked massive and cold. I got sick to my stomach and had this feeling of being swallowed by this structure. Each step we took toward the entrance felt heavier than the last. We walked through the front entrance, and I felt like we were being sucked inside, and I didn't know if we would ever be able to leave again. We had to go through the main lobby and begin the registration process. While we were sitting there, we ran into an acquaintance who had played basketball with my sister, Vicki. She, of course, wanted to know why we

DIAGNOSIS DAY

were there, and I left Mom to explain. I was still just going through the motions. Dick seemed to be holding up well, and I supposed he had to be strong for the rest of us.

We were first seen in the Pediatric Clinic at UIHC, where we registered at the desk and were asked to sit and wait for our names to be called. Alicia was in the play area that had a table and chairs, toys, and books. After what seemed like an eternity, but was only about 30 minutes, they called Alicia's name. We were taken to a room where we met the nurses. Mary Lou Linder, one of the oncology staff nurses, was our primary contact and such a wonderfully pleasant person. Alicia played with toys in the cupboard in that room while Mary Lou chatted and asked us questions about our family. She, too, had a daughter named Alicia. We discussed our daughter's medical history, including family medical history, and provided general health information.

With her small Raggedy Ann doll in tow, Alicia toddled down the hallway to the lab for the first of countless finger pokes. She sat on my lap, wincing only when the needle stuck her little finger. The lab was equipped with a variety of boo-boo strips, though, which seemed to make the poke less painful. I will always remember Alicia with her Raggedy Ann doll in tow—her constant companion—throughout her cancer journey. Just as with the finger poke, that doll appeared to bring Alicia comfort, which, in a small way, comforted me as well.

We met with Dr. Kisker, who ordered additional X-rays and scans. He told us we would be admitted and he'd be in later to tell us what they had learned from these additional tests. Alicia had been an exceptional girl. She smiled at everyone she met, and all the available toys intrigued her.

Several hours passed by the time we were through with the clinic and lab for blood work and were shown to our room. Alicia had a private room that shared the bathroom with the patient and his family in the next room. The nursing staff showed us around the floor, including the toy and waiting rooms. Just outside our room was a room with some supplies and a refrigerator. Out of that room appeared a little boy, the same age as Alicia. His name was Michael, and he was born with neuroblastoma. Michael's tumor was in his abdomen. He had a kidney removed shortly after birth. The cancer was in his bone marrow. All of this meant Michael had been in treatment since he was born, and now, at about two years of age, he had just a treatment or two to go and was doing well. What an inspiration that sweet child was. That moment provided me with more hope and optimism than I had in days. If he could look this good after a two-year battle, then we were going to give this disease a good fight, too!

So many of these children were an inspiration to us during this difficult time. I particularly remember a 5-year-old named Steven. He apparently had endured a day of high-endurance testing. I recall his dad saying to him, "Steven, we are so proud of you. You were so brave." Steven's immediate response was, "Oh, Dad, I know when you had to do this, you were brave." He just assumed everyone had to do testing. I had never thought that a 5-year-old would believe we had all gone through what he had and it was OK. It brought tears to my eyes and I had to walk away. But, make no mistake, I was inspired by his resolve.

When we got back to our room, my mom was standing in the doorway, talking to a pretty, tall, slim woman. She looked to be about my age, 30-ish, and had a worn, anxious look about her. She was obviously a parent. Mom was in tears, and this woman was trying to comfort her, telling her she knew what we were going through. Her name was Ladonna Czachowski, and she was there with her son Philip. Philip had been diagnosed on Mother's Day that year, and they had been in the hospital ever since. She truly did know what we were going through; it had only been a few weeks since she had learned about her son, Philip. We visited briefly, but it wasn't until later that evening that I had some time with Ladonna. I knew instantly we were going to be good friends.

DIAGNOSIS DAY

"I don't know how we are going to get through this, Ladonna," I told her.

"Oh, I know how you are feeling," she said. "You keep thinking you are going to wake up anytime now, and it will all have been a dream. You don't. You pick up the pieces, and you move forward for your child. A mother's instincts just kick in, and you do whatever it is that you need to do to protect and care for your child. No one can tell you how you are feeling. Even those of us who have walked the same path feel things differently."

"I'm glad you are our neighbor," I told Ladonna. "I'll probably be over there all the time with questions."

"You stop by anytime, Peggy," she told me. "And remember, we share a bathroom . . . backdoor guests are always best."

That moment made me feel like we were not in this alone. With swollen eyes and drained emotions, I knew I could, and would, come to depend on Ladonna.

II
LEARNING THE ROPES

Somehow, we made it through day one in the University of Iowa Hospitals and Clinics. We were introduced to countless staff, doctors and nurses. One in particular, "tall Jane," a floor nurse, was memorable because she made us all feel as comfortable as possible. My folks took a shine to her and always asked about her after subsequent hospital visits.

That first day, we also met a 3-year-old girl, who had her eyes removed because of tumors on them. She, too, was named Alicia. Her parents had been given 24 hours to decide between taking her eyes and having her survive or letting her keep her eyes and ultimately losing her battle with cancer. They decided to have the surgery. Thankfully, she survived surgery.

Fearing all the decisions we were going to have to make, the thought of taking someone's eyes so they could survive was unimaginable. Alicia's mom was a young, slightly built woman with short blonde hair. Meeting these kids and their parents was overwhelming, but I quickly realized we weren't in this alone, nor were we the only ones making tough decisions. How many sick kids are there???

Our introductory day at UIHC was emotionally draining, much like diagnosis day at Mercy Hospital. Afterwards, Dick went home to be with the boys and explain to them and his mom what little we had learned. My folks left to provide the same report to my other family members. We would be in for another long day tomorrow, and all needed some rest. I did not rest well as I repeatedly relived the events of the day, trying to comprehend everything the doctors told us — which wasn't much more than we already knew before we arrived at the UIHC — and to accept the fact that tomorrow would be another day of testing.

There was so much that kept me from sleeping. Earlier in the day, we met with an oncology nurse, who had given us information to read about neuroblastoma and treatment. I wanted all the information I could gather to read and try to understand. Yet, I couldn't concentrate on the material. I'd start reading, and then I'd cry, and I'd start over, and then I'd stand by Alicia's bed where she was coloring and playing. Then, I'd start reading again.

It was still hard to imagine that our little girl could be as sick as they said she was. We thought she had a cold. Maybe she had pneumonia, even tuberculosis. As strange as it sounds, at that exact moment, I wished it could have been any of those things. CANCER just seemed to be this overwhelmingly heavy, daunting word. Nothing happy or good ever seemed to me to come from it. I could not believe she was so sick when she looked to be such a picture of health. No one would have known, which is why we initially didn't suspect anything serious. I returned to reading and must have read the first page at least a dozen times. If someone had asked me what was on that first page, I would not have had a clue. What I do remember is that neuroblastoma is a childhood cancer that generally does not attack anyone over the age of 5, and was, at that time —more than 40 years ago now — a newer form of cancer. The available printed information, even for hospitals, was limited.

Alicia seemed pretty worn out from her tests and was ready for bed. She didn't appear afraid of the strange room or the bars on her bed and quickly settled in. Ladonna, from the room next door, got Philip settled in as well, and then we sat on the bathroom floor that our private rooms shared and chatted. I filled her in on what we believed we were up against, and she told me a little about their situation. Philip had been admitted, diagnosed, and started treatment, all within a week. They had already been there about six weeks, during which time their house was burglarized. Ladonna had not been home. She had stayed at Philip's side in the hospital, which I knew was exactly what I would do.

Our conversation was calming, almost serene. Neither of us dwelled on the "whys" and the "what for," but rather just what we faced. Although our children were fighting totally different battles, we were in the same boat. There was no longer the need to explain how we felt or why we needed to cry.

I can't tell you how many times someone would say, "I know just how you feel." NO, you can't possibly know how I feel unless you are the parent of a child with a life-threatening illness! I appreciated people trying to help and trying to know the right thing to say. However, at that point, there was no right thing to say. Short of someone telling you this has all been a bad dream and there is nothing wrong with your child, there is no right thing. The doctors and nurses can't know, regardless of the training they have received or the number of times they have been through a diagnosis. Grandparents, aunts, uncles, cousins, good friends… just don't know. People can empathize with you and share your worry, but can't truly know HOW you feel.

I didn't sleep well that night, but at least I could stay in Alicia's room, so I was close to her. The floor we were on was bright, clean and quiet. I slept on a couch next to her bed.

Alicia was up and ready to play the next morning. She ate some of her breakfast and then wanted to find the toys. We went to the playroom for a while, until it was time for more tests. She was again sedated for a bone scan in nuclear medicine. She would never have laid still if she had not had the sedation. I wheeled her to the scan in a stainless-steel cart with sides designed to keep her from falling out. It didn't look very comfortable, but Alicia didn't complain and fell asleep on the way. I sat and looked at a magazine while she was in the test, only the pictures, since I couldn't concentrate on reading anything. There were also more X-rays. If you have ever had to sit in a hospital waiting for tests to be done, you know what it is like. I have never spent so much time waiting in my life. And as we came to discover, this was only the beginning of the waiting game.

Once the bone scan was finished and the X-rays taken, we headed back to Alicia's room. She needed to sleep off the sedation, so I started writing a few notes to friends I was sure would want to know we were in the hospital. Writing these notes and putting what I knew into words made the diagnosis seem truer and clearer.

Alicia's "primary" nurse was Denise, a young woman who was kind and gentle. Affectionately known to us as "Neece," she was with us the entire time of treatment. If we were in the hospital for treatment and Neece was working, she was assigned to us. Some 20 years later, we found Denise to be part of the Neo-Natal Department, and just recently, I saw her at the hospital just days prior to her retirement.

Dick came back to the hospital after work. I talked to him numerous times during the day to keep him abreast of what we were doing and what tests were being run. I know it was hard on him not to be at the hospital, but we also knew he would not be able to sit and wait like I was doing for the next tests and results. He needed to continue working, and I knew he was just a phone call away if we needed him. There wasn't anything to do but sit and wait. When he got to the hospital, we discussed the day's activities, and I told him what a good girl he had and how brave she was. By this time, Alicia was awake and ready to play again, so we all returned to the toy room.

After a while, we headed back to Alicia's room because we knew her supper would be coming soon. We ran into Dr. Kisker in the hallway. Balding and, I'm guessing, in his late 30s, and of course, wearing a white coat, Dr. Kisker was a straightforward and honest, but gentle man. We never had to wonder what he wasn't telling us; he just laid it all out. This evening, he had results from some of the tests.

I'm not sure why we stood in the hallway instead of going to Alicia's room, but I recall standing there listening intently to his every word. He began by stating his diagnosis was the same as Dr. Hackbarth's. Yes, Alicia has neuroblastoma. Her tumor was very large and behind her heart. They had not found tumors anywhere else in her body, and the cancer had not invaded her bone marrow. Those findings were extremely good news. Dr. Kisker indicated he would give us a 50-50 chance, and that was only because Alicia's tumor was in her chest. With neuroblastoma, children with tumors in their chest had a better survival rate than those with abdominal tumors. I don't think I ever asked why. I guess I was just relieved to be in the higher survival category. My response to Dr. Kisker was, "OK . . . we'll take the 50-50 and fight as hard as we possibly can!" Dr. Kisker also mentioned the possibility of surgery but told us he would be in later to discuss that in greater detail.

Dick and I took Alicia back to her room and got her ready for supper. I had packed some food and brought it from home for myself or whoever was staying at the hospital with Alicia. I knew the expense of eating hospital food would become immense if we were going to be at this for any length of time. I brought in a few basics I knew would get us through, such as crackers, popcorn, cheese, and veggies. Grandma and Grandpa had made it clear they would bring something to share when they visited, and I knew Dick could bring food when he came up. Alicia often wanted the food from Grandma and Grandpa or from home, while the caregiver — usually me — was blessed with the hospital food.

Dick and I discussed Dr. Kisker's visit while Alicia ate supper. I think there was a sense of relief for both of us. Knowing what we were up against was more reassuring than not knowing. We still had no idea exactly what we were in for or how long the road would be, but we had a diagnosis, and we had ruled out tumors in other parts of her little body. We both knew we still had no control over what was ahead, but a diagnosis was at least a place to start.

After making the rest of his rounds, as promised, Dr. Kisker returned to discuss surgery. He said that because of the size of Alicia's tumor, the oncologists felt we needed to go in and surgically remove or "debulk" as much of the tumor as possible. Assuming we would agree, the surgery had been scheduled for the next day. Although there was no chance of removing the entire tumor, the doctors thought they had to remove as much tumor as possible and fight the rest with chemotherapy and radiation. Dr. Loren Hiratzka, our thoracic surgeon, arrived to explain the procedure and reassure us they would take as much tumor as possible to make our fight easier. The surgeons would enter through Alicia's back, with the incision starting about the middle of her back, going around her shoulder blade, and over to her left side. Dr. Hiratzka explained the risks and cautioned us the surgery would take at least 8 hours. Next, the anesthesiologist appeared in Alicia's room to explain procedures, risks and to answer our questions. We listened and signed release forms, hoping and praying we were doing the right thing. We were putting every ounce of faith and trust in people we didn't know. However, we didn't really think we had many choices, either. So, surgery it was.

The next morning came quickly. Alicia could not eat or drink anything, so we visited the toy room for a while to help entertain her and keep her from thinking about eating. Dick arrived, and while we watched Alicia play, we again expressed our hope that we were doing the right thing by putting her through surgery. Grandma Timm was keeping the boys again. We were so lucky to have her in Tipton and willing and able to help.

My folks arrived, and Dick and I took Alicia back to her room so they could start prepping her for surgery. Someone started an IV, injecting medications into it to make Alicia sleepy. Our pastor was on vacation, but he had arranged for Chaplain Lee from the UIHC to come and be with us. Chaplain Lee was a tall, wonderfully calming man, who came to Alicia's room and prayed with us before her surgery. When they came to take Alicia to surgery, the nurses told me I could walk with her part of the way. I thought that was a wonderful idea until we got to the elevator, and they told me I'd have to leave her. I gave her a hug and a kiss and told her I loved her. I didn't break down and cry until the elevator doors closed. That was the most horrid feeling I'd ever had. As the doors slowly closed, I wondered if I'd ever see my daughter alive again. They took her away, and I had no idea where the operating room was or what big, cold room she was going to be in all by herself.

I went back to her room to gather Dick, my parents, the chaplain, and something to read or do for the next eight hours. We were directed to the surgical waiting room and picked out a corner we thought would be comfortable for the duration of our stay. There was the usual coffee pot, teapot, and pop machine. We all just sat there, looking at each other. There wasn't anything to say. We had not been there too long when my lifelong friend, Barb Male, joined us. I was glad to see her, not because I thought she could provide comfort, but because we'd been friends so long, and I didn't feel the need to talk. She could imagine how I felt.

I couldn't read or work on the cross-stitching I had with me, so I just sat there looking out the window or staring at the door to the hallway. In less than one hour, the surgeon came through the door and headed to our cubicle. My heart sank. Nothing he had to say could be good news. We had been told to prepare for a long, 8-hour surgery, after which someone would come to tell us the results. This had been less than 60 minutes! What could have happened? Was she still alive? Were they postponing surgery? It was amazing how many questions ran through my mind in the few seconds it took the surgeon to cross the room.

He sat down in a chair next to Dick, facing me, and started with, "Your daughter is fine. She is in recovery." The tumor was too large for them to even start the debulking process.

"There isn't a blood vessel in or out of her heart that isn't tangled in tumor. So, we had to close and will have to try chemotherapy first. There was no possibility of taking a portion of the tumor without other risks," he explained. I was somewhat disheartened, but perhaps sensing our anxiety, the surgeon quickly continued, telling us that closing and leaving the tumor intact was not all bad. The tumor appeared to be a solid mass; leaving it intact seemed a better option than trying to cut away at it. They did, however, take a small piece that would be sent to Los Angeles, where they were doing a significant amount of neuroblastoma research, for a complete biopsy report. Alicia would be in recovery for a short time and then back down on the floor, where we could see her.

Finally, the surgeon outlined the plan going forward: Once Alicia had a couple of days to recover from her surgery, chemotherapy would start. She would receive the cancer chemotherapy drugs Cytoxan, DTIC, and Vincristine at the beginning of her 92-week protocol. 92 weeks! In the beginning, I couldn't even comprehend how long 92 weeks were. When it finally sank in and I announced that 92 weeks was almost two years, I seemed to be the only one surprised by that revelation. 92 weeks. That was more weeks of chemotherapy and radiation than Alicia had been alive. One of the nurses told me that I shouldn't think of it in terms of 92 weeks. I should take it one week at a time, which would help everyone cope better. In very short order, I learned not even to count weeks but to take one day at a time. Hell, sometimes you must take half days and pray to get through those!

Alicia's chemotherapy started on July 9. Even with nausea medicine, she got very sick to her stomach. Cytoxan was the drug that made her the sickest. We were told Alicia would likely get sick for about three hours after administration of the Cytoxan, which she received via a pump. After just two rounds of chemo, when the nursing staff arrived with the pump, Alicia knew exactly what was about to happen. Throughout her entire treatment, we could set our watches, 30 minutes after the pump was started, she would vomit. And vomit and vomit. Generally, the vomiting would subside in about three hours, and she could sleep. She would sleep three hours, then be ready to stroll the halls and play in the toy room.

Alicia would get chemotherapy for five days. We would go home for two weeks and then return to the hospital for five more days of chemo. Looking back at that schedule and having the boys at home, I have no idea how we managed to endure it. It was certainly not without the help and support of friends, neighbors, and family.

Walking the halls and going to play in the toy room was a bit of a challenge with a toddler hooked to an IV pole for medications and hydration. As Alicia's veins were used repeatedly, it became harder and harder to find good veins. Alicia's IV could be unhooked for a while to make her more mobile, and the infusion site would be protected by a medical "device," generally a Styrofoam cup taped over the site, so the IV could be restarted at any time.

Other than Alicia's nausea, the first round of chemo had gone pretty well. Upon completing her first five days, we went home, hoping to return to some form of normalcy. I know now that "normalcy" was not possible. But if Alicia's blood counts were good in two weeks, we would be back for round 2. With the tests at Mercy and the tests, surgery, and chemo at the UIHC, we had been in the hospital for three weeks. I was ready to be home with the boys.

The return for round 2, of course, meant making arrangements for the boys again. The boys were shuffled between grandparents, aunts, uncles, and friends. Again, I have no idea how we would have made it through this experience without the support of family and friends. Dick worked during the week, and I stayed at the hospital. On weekends, Dick stayed at the hospital, and I worked and went home to the boys. Because Alicia had to be hydrated before starting her chemo, we generally went in on Wednesday afternoon for any tests that needed to be done, including blood work and chest X-rays. They would start her IV, and then we would do chemo Thursday through Monday. If all went well, we could go home on Monday afternoon.

One morning, after Alicia's second round of chemo, while combing her hair, I realized Alicia was losing her shoulder-length strawberry blonde hair. I put a little green drop-waist dress on her that my mother had made for me when I was a child and took her to have her picture taken. Mom had made matching dresses for my sister Vicki and me for a cousin's wedding. I loved that little dress, now 30 years old, and I wanted a picture of Alicia in it with her hair! So, away we went to Iowa City to have her picture taken.

It was also after round 2 that we noticed Alicia falling more often. I called the pediatric oncology clinic and was told this was likely due to the drug Vincristine, which causes "drop foot" and weakness in the legs. She was probably stumbling over her own feet, causing her to fall. She always got up and started out again, but we noticed she was falling more and more frequently.

After a few days of watching her mobility worsen, we also realized her motor skills were decreasing. In a matter of days, she was unable to walk at all, and her hands were shaking. After several calls to the clinic, they decided we had better see the oncologists and check things out. They were still fairly certain these symptoms were side effects of the chemotherapy, maybe even a viral infection, and that we should watch her closely.

CHILDHOOD CANCER

In a matter of a few more days, and before we could get her back to the clinic, Alicia's condition worsened until she lost all her motor skills. She could no longer walk, crawl, sit, or hold a spoon to feed herself. She shook even when being held, and her eyes would bounce around in her little head. It was like she had no balance and could not focus.

I called the clinic again. I was so afraid of what was happening to Alicia and wanted them to observe her. We went into the clinic and were admitted. The oncologists feared the tumor had probably grown and was affecting her spinal column. A myelogram, which injected a dye to look for problems in the spinal canal, was scheduled for the next day to see if the tumor was affecting her spine.

While putting the dye in Alicia's veins, a vein burst, and the dye infiltrated the tissue in the back of her hand, burning it very badly. When the myelogram was finished, we had to keep her lying flat on her back for several hours. This chore, coupled with having to tie her hand to the bed above her head so the dye would not drain out of her hand and into the rest of her system, was no small feat. The good thing was they did not find tumor on her spinal column. The downside is her left hand is much smaller than her right, and she has very poor circulation in her burnt hand. It is always cold and hurts when the weather turns cold. The doctor administering the dye convinced me the burn was just an accident. I now wish I had pursued the issue. I think someone wasn't paying attention when the dye was being administered, or it may have been stopped. Oh, hindsight. At that particular moment, I thought we had more crucial issues, and that there wasn't tumor on her spine was great news. We, however, did not have any answers as to what was causing her balance problems.

The tests seemed to be continuous. I can't even count the number of CAT scans, MRIs, bone scans, bone marrow scans, and X-rays taken, and the amount of blood drawn from her little body for tests. We did some of these at all times of the day and night, whenever the equipment was available.

We had to do another 24-hour urine collection to test her dopamine. To do so, we had to put a bag on her. This procedure worked for a few hours with the adhesive on the bag, but midway into the urine collection, as the bag got wet, it always seemed to me that the nursing staff had to use a stronger adhesive resembling super glue. I felt so sorry for Alicia, but she never complained, and we always managed to get through it. Only a couple of times did the bag let go completely, and we'd have to start all over. Those incidents were extremely frustrating. I was thrilled when she was potty-trained and could pee in a "hat" on the stool for collection.

After a couple more days of tests, the doctors decided Alicia's system was fighting the tumor so hard that the chemical imbalance was causing the shakiness and motor skill loss she was experiencing. So, another scan in nuclear medicine was scheduled, as well as chest X-rays, to decide if a second surgery was a viable option.

I remember taking Alicia to the nuclear medicine department in the small stainless-steel cart used to transport infants and toddlers. We fondly referred to them as the "little tin beds." Alicia and I had grown very fond of a nuclear medicine technician named Tony. He was always kind, gentle, and compassionate, and seemed to calm Alicia just by talking to her and assuring her that he would stay with her. Meanwhile, I would sit in the waiting room during her scan, trying to distract myself with a magazine. In all the hours I sat and waited, I never learned how to manage my stress or stay interested in anything. I couldn't concentrate. I tried reading, writing, and cross-stitching. Nothing could ever hold my interest or attention.

The assisting thoracic surgeon from Alicia's first surgery came in and sat beside me.

"Are you here with Alicia Timm?" he asked.

"Yes," I replied, anxious about the question.

"What are the oncologists thinking?" he asked.

Although puzzled by his questions, I answered: "They are considering surgery to see if they can take some of the tumor. Her little body is fighting the tumor so hard that it has her entire system out of kilter."

I had no idea where he was going with his question or why he seemed so indignant. He went on . . . "They are going to kill that little girl if they go back in there now. These oncologists were not in the original surgery. I was in there, and there is no way they can go back in without killing her."

I just sat there. I was numb. The oncologists were saying we needed to consider surgery to save her, and the assistant thoracic surgeon was saying she'd die if they went back in. I did not know what to do, so I sat in that waiting room, crying and reliving that conversation. Finally, they brought Alicia back to me in her tin tub, and we went back to her room.

Apparently, someone in nuclear medicine overheard my conversation with the assisting thoracic surgeon and alerted someone in hematology/oncology. We had hardly returned to our room when Dr. Raymond Tannous, another pediatric oncologist, arrived to apologize for the incident involving the thoracic surgeon. He went further to assure me that the oncologists, who reviewed Alicia's new scans, strongly suggested surgery after the two rounds of chemotherapy shrank the tumor away from Alicia's heart and blood vessels. He finished his visit by telling me it was up to us if we wanted the assisting surgeon back in the operating room for the second surgery. Our primary surgeon was out of town. As much as he had upset me, I decided that if he was good, and he had been highly recommended, he could be of help having been there for the first surgery. I wanted him there.

III
HOSPITAL LIFE

There were many more days of testing — all kinds of testing. One day, we had a scan scheduled. They gave Alicia sedation, but she did not go to sleep. Since she had been given so much sedation in the past couple of months, the staff decided to try Valium. It was stronger, just different, for her body. When that didn't help, the intern ordered a little more Valium.

I was holding and rocking Alicia. Although she only weighed 21 pounds, she was difficult to hold because of her body spasms. My mother was there that day. She asked, "Alicia, if Grandma holds you and rocks you, will you try to go to sleep?"

Alicia sat up and looked at Grandma. Despite her erratic eye movements, which affected her ability to focus on anything or anyone, she nodded her semi-bald head yes and reached for Grandma. Grandma took Alicia and moved to the rocking chair. She, too, was unsuccessful in getting Alicia to sleep . . . more sedation followed. The more sedation they gave her, the more high-strung she became. Alicia was not going to sleep.

I finally said, "No more! NO MORE!! I don't know how much Valium is too much, but I don't want her to have any more!" I don't know how much more Valium or other sedation the intern would have tried pushing, but I could see we were not headed in the right direction. This scan was going to have to be postponed and rescheduled. I'd be the first to admit my medical knowledge is limited, but parents know their children, and this was not working.

The same intern came to change the tubing on Alicia's IV pole. She stood bedside briefly, looked at me, and asked, "Do you know what size tubing they use for Alicia's IVs?"

Rather dumbfounded, I looked at her, "Uh, no, I have no idea."

"OK," she said. "I guess I better go find out before I start. It appears to be small."

I watched her leave the room. Although I said nothing, I thought, "Yeah, you better go find out now that we know you don't have a clue what you're doing!" Isn't this why every patient has notes and files at the nurse's station for reference? Alicia's file ultimately became a library.

Back she came with the knowledge she apparently needed and strung new lines on Alicia's IV pole. Later, I told one of the staff doctors we did not want that intern to be in Alicia's room or on her case. I added something ugly, like, "I thought her time would be better spent shoveling pig shit or snow, but in any event, I didn't think medical school was the best career choice for her."

Second Surgery Day

September 7 was the day set for Alicia's second major surgery. The surgeons were going back in to remove as much of the tumor as possible. They would re-enter right over the first set of scars from Alicia's original surgery. The oncologists were fairly convinced this was the only way to "re-balance" Alicia's system. Her little body was struggling so hard to fight the cancer that her entire system had become unbalanced, causing the spasms and jerking movements. The hope was enough tumor could

HOSPITAL LIFE

be removed so that her system would level out and her balance and motor skills would improve.

The thought of sending her back into surgery was daunting. My fear of the surgery was compounded by the assisting surgeon's comments after Alicia's first surgery, which kept running through my mind. In all honesty, however, I knew we didn't have much choice. Alicia was worsening by the day. Her ability to communicate or maneuver was declining rapidly. She could not be still lying in a bed or on the floor. She shook continually, her limbs jerked constantly, and her beautiful brown eyes bounced around her head like dice on a table. She couldn't focus, and her small hands could not grab or hold anything. She couldn't even suck her thumb because she couldn't hold it still. I was afraid of dropping her because of her body spasms.

A day or so before her second surgery, Alicia grabbed my necklace and broke the chain, which held the cross I had been wearing since the day she was diagnosed. Before that day, I had only worn my cross on special occasions: weddings, baptisms, family gatherings. Since Alicia's diagnosis, I decided we needed all the help we could get. So, I put my cross on, and although I have had to replace the chain numerous times, it has remained around my neck day and night since Diagnosis Day. I truly believe it helped me cope with Alicia's battle. It has certainly been a comfort to me. I hold it regularly, sometimes with prayer and sometimes to count my blessings.

I had come to terms with the fact that Alicia's situation was out of our hands. We could love, care for, and support her, but ultimately, her survival was out of our hands. We had no control. The doctors, the nurses, and family members were caregivers. Whether she survived was not up to us.

A new intern told me he thought she needed a swat on her butt after she'd broken my chain. One of the staff oncologists interjected, he thought she was acting out of frustration and needed to be held tight to know she was loved. He explained, we should think of her behavior in terms of how we would feel if we had gone from walking and talking to being unable to do either, and instead having someone do everything for us. It was much the same for her. Alicia had gone from being a walking, talking, almost-2-year-old to someone who couldn't sit, crawl, or hold her spoon. This made perfect sense to me, so we sat and rocked her, hugged her, and loved her.

Dick came to the hospital after getting off work. We had been inpatients for several days before surgery by this time. This evening, we had to meet with the surgeon and anesthesiologist to review the procedures, sign forms — again — and ask last-minute questions. We didn't have many questions. In this situation, it is difficult to even think of questions you should ask. I guess they had done as good a job as possible explaining what would take place.

Dick didn't stay too long at the hospital. He wanted to spend some time with the boys and would be back in the morning before surgery.

The boys seemed to be doing well with all the changes in their lives. At this point, they were spending most of their time with Grandma Timm. And because school had started, they needed to be in the school district.

Morning dawned, and the day for surgery had arrived. Like the last time, Alicia couldn't have anything to eat or drink. We closed her room door so she wouldn't see the breakfast trays being delivered. She was content being held and rocked. When she was tired of being in her bed, she couldn't sit by herself, and I couldn't lay her on the uncarpeted floor for fear she'd hurt her head thrashing around. So, I held her, and I sang along to Sesame Street on the television.

This was one of the first times I admitted to myself that I was tiring. We were only about 10 weeks into this diagnosis, and I was wearing out. I didn't let anyone else know. I needed to be strong. But what I was feeling this morning was different. There had been so many days since diagnosis — tests, test results, reports, and waiting — I was just plain tired. I felt physically and emotionally drained. The tears came easily when there was quiet time. The roller coaster ride had been a challenge, and for a brief moment, I just wanted off. Not having that option, I took a long, hard look around her room, took some deep breaths, and decided to be as strong as I could be for Alicia.

Her surgery was scheduled for late morning, and time seemed to stand still. Pastor Franker and my parents joined Dick and me at the hospital. At about 9:30 that morning, the nurse gave Alicia medicine to make her drowsy, and we rocked. When it was time for surgery, I placed her on the big transport cart, covered her with a warm blanket, kissed her, and told her we loved her and would be waiting for her to return to us. The nurse offered me the option of going as far as the elevators with Alicia, but remembering the first such offer, I declined, choosing to stay in her room instead. They took my baby off to surgery one more time. She looked so fragile and vulnerable in that big bed. They were barely out of the door when my tears started to flow. I was even more worried about this surgery than the first because I knew they had to be able to help her this time. I didn't know if there would be additional opportunities for surgery. I kept hearing the surgeon's comments: "They will kill that little girl if they go back in."

We were all more tired, worn out, and emotionally drained than we were for the first surgery. Pastor Franker was so good to us. We sat in Alicia's semi-dark room for a few minutes, giving me time to regroup, and then we all held hands and prayed together for our little girl. We prayed for everyone to be granted the strength needed to get through the day. After a few more minutes, we gathered our belongings and busy work and headed for the surgical waiting room.

We checked in at the waiting room desk and settled in for the long haul. I picked a quiet corner where we would be somewhat isolated. I remember people — family and friends — coming and going, and Dick pacing. He went to get something cold to drink. I just sat, staring into space or at the door to our waiting room. I wasn't expecting anyone, I just stared. I couldn't get interested in or concentrate on anything. After quite a while, we were told surgery had started.

"Started?" I asked with surprise. "I thought they would have been well into the process by now."

"Well, no," the staff person assured me. "Preparation for surgery takes some time, and if they had to wait for an operating room or a surgeon, the start time is often delayed. They are started now, however, and we'll let you know as soon as they are finished."

Although it seemed like a lifetime, surgery took less time than predicted. Four hours after surgery began, the waiting room volunteer told us the surgeon would be out shortly to speak with us. In a few minutes, I saw him coming through the door. Dr. Brandt, whose first name I can't remember, as there were so many medical professionals you lose track, was tall, seemingly much too young to be a surgeon. All sorts of thoughts were racing through my mind as he crossed the short distance to where we were sitting.

He seemed calm and sat down in a chair facing me. Dick was standing off to the side where he could hear. I don't think he'd sat down the entire time.

"Alicia handled the surgery very well," Dr. Brandt began. "She had no problems with the procedure, and I have good news. I am fairly certain we have been able to take the entire tumor."

"Really?" I know I sounded shocked. My chin dropped in disbelief. "I can't believe you were able to take most, if not all, of the tumor." Immediately, the relief tears flowed. I reached for Dick's hand, and he squeezed mine.

"With just two rounds of chemotherapy, amazingly, the tumor shrank away from her heart, and the blood vessels that were the major concern in the first surgery were more visible," Dr. Brandt continued. "The tumor seems to be self-contained. However, we took tissue surrounding the tumor to biopsy and make sure we didn't miss any diseased cells. The surrounding tissue will be sent to Los Angeles again for testing."

"OK," I sighed with relief. "Now, what do we do?"

"As soon as Alicia has had some recovery time, the oncologists will likely continue with her protocol," said Dr. Brandt. "She's a strong little girl, but her body will require some days to heal. She has just been through major surgery. She will be in the ICU for a couple of days, and then, if all goes well, she will be transferred back down to her unit. Depending on how she recovers, she will either be sent to the intermediate ICU on the second floor or directly back to her room.

"Do you have any other questions?" he asked.

We did not. He told us Dick and I could see Alicia for a few minutes once she was moved to the ICU.

"Thank you," Dick continued, with relief in his voice. "If we have any questions, will someone from ICU know how to get in touch with you?"

"Absolutely," Dr. Brandt responded. "I will be back to check on Alicia a little later and update you. Let staff know if you leave the area."

The air in the waiting room seemed lighter. You could feel the relief in all of us. The road was still going to be long and potentially bumpy, but this was exceptional news!

The waiting room attendant indicated it would be some time before Alicia would be moved from recovery to ICU, so if we wanted to get food or go for a walk, we should do so.

I thanked the attendant, whose red hair was obviously not natural, and told her we would be back in an hour.

The thought of taking a walk and getting something cold to drink was appealing. But I could not move. I was running Dr. Brandt's words through my mind again and again. We were extremely thankful Alicia had survived another surgery and were hopeful they had been able to take the entire tumor. That was wonderful news we didn't even hope for. I started to cry.

"Are you OK?" asked Pastor Franker. He looked around the room to gather support from those who knew me best. "I don't know what to do here. She cries when she's sad, and she cries when she's happy!"

"I'm fine," I said to him through tears. "It is such a relief to have Alicia out of surgery, alive and recovering. The entire tumor being removed is almost more than I can comprehend. I hope the lab results from her biopsy are as encouraging."

We gathered our belongings and headed to Alicia's room. She would not be returning to this room for a couple of days, but I intended to stay all night, and this is likely where I'd try to get some sleep.

After we unloaded our junk in her room and checked in at the nurses' station, I wanted to go right back up to the ICU waiting room. Just in case we could see Alicia, I wanted to be there. Dick knew enough to agree. I told him I should go back to ICU, and he would get something cold to drink and bring it to me.

Knowing visitors in ICU would be limited, Pastor headed home to his family, and my parents left to report our excellent news to the rest of our family. My folks were retired from 40-plus years of farming. Spending days in the hospital must have been very long and stressful for them. I'm sure they were tired and ready for some rest.

I went upstairs to the ICU waiting room. Soon, Dick joined me with cold drinks in hand.

We hadn't been sitting there for too long when one of the nurses came and told us we could go in to see Alicia. I could tell from the look on Dick's face this moment had come quicker than he had anticipated. He just did not want to go to the ICU. He turned ashen gray. Despite his large frame and robust stature, he looked vulnerable and weak. ICU is where he had seen his dad for the last time before he died of cancer. It took every ounce of strength that man could muster to walk through those doors. I knew he wanted to see his little girl, and I was hoping he'd have some peace of mind by seeing her recovering.

Dick was in there for a very short time. Long enough to touch her, tell her he loved her, and then he was back out the door. It was all a little overwhelming. ICU was very cold and very bright.

I stood at Alicia's bedside, watching her sleep peacefully. There were monitors beeping and sterile stainless steel everywhere. Her heart monitor was beeping regularly. I assume one was for blood pressure. She seemed so tiny in the big bed. Not a stitch of clothes on her. A tube was coming out of almost every opening in her little body. There was a tube in her nose. There was a tube down her throat. There was a drainage tube in her neck, one in her side, and one to collect her urine connected to a bag hanging on the side of her bed. I remember thinking there was more equipment and tubing than she was big.

One of the nurses came over to Alicia's bed. "She's doing very well, Mom." She continued, "We have to ask you to keep your visits short, but you are welcome to come back later and sit with her again. If you are going to be in the ICU waiting room, we can come and get you if there is any change in her condition."

Comfortable with that, I went back to the ICU waiting room to find Dick. I knew by looking at him I would not get him to go back in there. I never asked him to. He had been in to see his girl and told her he loved her. That was enough.

After a short time in the ICU waiting room, Dick headed home. Grandma Timm, widowed young and left with children to raise, was now retired from the UIHC food service. She was so good to the boys. I'm sure she was exhausted by the end of most days after caring for the boys, but she never complained. Dick intended to work the next day, and this one had been exhausting for all of us. I walked him downstairs to the lobby. We stood and relived parts of the day. We were encouraged by Alicia's surgery.

"I think we're pretty lucky," I said. "I think someone was watching over us and answered some prayers for us today."

"I think you're absolutely right," Dick said. "I know we still have a long road ahead, but this has been a good day."

He gave me a hug and a kiss and said, "I'm going home to spend some time with our boys. Let me know if there are any changes in Alicia's condition. Otherwise, I'll wait to hear from you in the morning about what kind of night she had."

"OK, see you tomorrow," I said. "Get home safe, give the boys big hugs, and tell them I love them. Get some sleep."

I didn't want him to leave, but I knew it was better for the boys and Dick. Just as he was leaving, Vonnie walked into the hospital. She just got off work. She had gone to work after losing Loren five years earlier. I can't imagine what I would have done without the love and support of our families. Too many families have to go through this alone or with family hundreds of miles away. We were so lucky to have ours close.

"Well, hi, little sister," she said, surprised to see me in the lobby. "How is Alicia? How are you?"

"Hi, Vonnie. I'm fine, and Alicia is good." I relayed our good news to her.

"Great!" she said. "The hospital is not my first choice in places to spend my birthday, but if the news is good, it makes it much easier!"

"Oh, I'm sorry!" Giving her a hug for her birthday and for being supportive, I said, "I forgot it was your birthday. Happy Birthday, Sweet Sister!"

Before, I had started to wonder if I would come to dislike the 7th of any month since July 7th was Alicia's first surgery and her second surgery

HOSPITAL LIFE

was September 7th. Not anymore. Vonnie's birthday being September 7th was a good omen!

"It's OK," she assured me. "Not like you didn't have some more important things on your mind. I'm so pleased you got good, maybe even great news!"

Vonnie and I sat in a couple of chairs in the lobby. I knew I wouldn't be allowed back in to see Alicia yet and wanted a change of scenery. The lobby, at least, provided a diverse mix of people and décor. We talked more about the day and Alicia's surgery. A few more tears were shed in relief and thankfulness. I knew we weren't out of the woods, but a day like this was encouraging enough to help us get through the next few. You find yourself hanging on to the littlest signs and faintest rays of hope. This day and the news we had received provided much reassurance. Our roller coaster car seemed to be climbing again.

Vonnie and I sat there, talking, crying, laughing. Our laughter was triggered by just watching people. We got tickled when part of The University of Iowa football team shuffled through the hospital's main lobby after football practice at the nearby football field. They were on their way back to their dorms, most of them plodding along with untied shoes. We decided the trainers didn't have time to help them tie their sneakers. That shared thought—likely only funny to us—produced gales of whispered laughter.

A little more time passed, and a group of six or eight people sat down not far from us. They all wore shirts in a golden-brown color with their names on them.

"That must be a bowling team that stopped off to see a friend in the hospital," said Vonnie.

I broke into hysterical laughter. She looked at me like I'd lost my mind, and I said, "Vonnie, that is the housekeeping personnel for the hospital.

That's why they all have matching shirts. Let's assume they are just taking a break!"

We have repeatedly laughed about that conversation since. It felt so good to laugh. I truly did not remember the last time I laughed out loud. The news that day was encouraging, but you can ask anyone who has been through illnesses like these . . . you are ALWAYS guarded. Your life becomes such a roller coaster that you are almost afraid to let your guard down. You're afraid to become hopeful or optimistic. You're afraid to think positively because you know someone might come in and deliver bad news that will again bring you crashing down as quickly as good news provides you with hope and faith.

I wanted to go back to the ICU just in case they would let me see Alicia again. We walked slowly across the lobby, down the never-ending hallways, and took the elevator back to the ICU waiting room. Finally, I was able to see Alicia again. Vonnie could not go with me, but I was going to see my girl! Alicia was still sleeping so peacefully, which I knew was good for her. I just wanted to wrap her in a warm blanket and hold her close. She looked so tiny and helpless. She was such a pretty little thing, so precious to her mom. There were still tubes and monitors everywhere. I stroked her arm and forehead and told her how much I loved her. Then I went back to the waiting room, where I'd wait until the next time I got permission to have a few more minutes with her.

Vonnie decided to head home. She'd been at work all day, had kids at home, and hadn't had dinner. I walked her back down to the main lobby and the entrance door.

She hugged me and said, "You hang in there! Give Alicia hugs from her Aunt Vonnie when you can and tell her we are all keeping her in our prayers."

"I will," I said. "And Happy Birthday. I'm really sorry I forgot."

"It's OK. You just take care of things here, and we'll celebrate all these good things sometime soon."

"OK, get home safe. Your sister loves you!"

"Your sister loves you, too," she said. "Get some rest when you can."

I watched my oldest sister walk out the front doors. She had some rough years after losing her husband, Loren, and having kids to raise. We had our share of disagreements in prior years. Vonnie is 12 years older than I am, and for many years, I did not think she particularly liked her little sister. I was more of an annoyance she had to help take care of. She particularly remembers having to iron my pinafores and pretty dresses when she would rather have been outside. Thankfully, she — we — were past all of that.

I returned to the ICU waiting room and checked in. Knowing it would be a while before I could see Alicia again, I settled into a chair with a magazine. I couldn't concentrate. I spent the next few hours alternating between a chair and a couch that was far too short for my long legs. They let me into the ICU a couple more times to see Alicia and then suggested I go to her room to sleep. I could come up as soon as I was up in the morning or anytime during the night if I was awake. They would take good care of her and call if there was any change in her condition. They assured me she and I both needed sleep. I was really tired. I'd already fallen asleep a couple of times on the uncomfortable couch. So, I returned to the second floor and tried to get settled in there. I knew she wasn't far away, and I knew there was nothing I could do for her. Nonetheless, I had trouble getting comfortable. I re-lived the day, the conversations, and how Alicia looked in that big, cold bed. I must have finally drifted off because it was daylight when I came to. Without showering or getting ready for the day, I went right back up to the ICU.

The nursing staff said she'd had a good night and that she was a fighter. She had pulled her nose tube out in the middle of the night. It did not seem it would have to be reinserted, which they said was a good sign of

Alicia's healing. Alicia knew she was through with the tube and eliminated it. That, again, was encouraging. I knew she was an independent, headstrong little girl, and this just proved it.

The ICU staff sent me back to Alicia's room to rest, assuring me they would let me know of any change. I obeyed. I reached her room and called Dick to give him an early morning report. "Alicia had a good night and even took out one of her tubes," I told Dick. "She is still sleeping and has been all night. They must be giving her something for pain and to keep her quiet."

"That's good. Did you sleep?" Dick asked me.

"I did, once I got to sleep," I told him. "It must have been between midnight and 1 a.m., but I slept until daylight. I might need to work in a nap sometime later today if Alicia is doing all right."

"That would be a good idea," Dick said.

"How are the boys?" I asked.

"They are fine. They were glad to hear their sister is doing better. I'm not sure how much either of them really understands about all this surgery," Dick said. "I know Tony better understands how sick Alicia is than Andy. It's all confusing to them, however.

"Oh, I know. It's confusing to all of us! Did you sleep?" I asked him.

"Yeah, but not very well," he said. "I kept thinking about the surgeons' comments and hoping that they really were able to get all of the tumor."

"I know," I said. "Vonnie and I think we'll have to find time to celebrate. She was here just after you left last night and stayed for a couple of hours. It was her birthday."

"Well," said Dick, "I guess I'll see you after work. If you need me to come over for any reason, just let me know."

"OK, talk to you later. Bye."

HOSPITAL LIFE

The patient's rooms had shower and bath facilities that parents could use. I showered, got cleaned up, and then returned to the ICU waiting room. I had just gone back in to see Alicia when a friend of ours, who worked in security at the hospital, stopped by. They let him come to her bedside. Seeing someone I knew besides medical staff in white coats was so good. He was very encouraging, telling me how good she looked. She did look good. Her color was better.

She still looked small in the bed, wired and connected by tubes, but she was starting to become more alert, and it was great to see those pretty brown eyes again.

By noon, less than 24 hours post-surgery, they transferred Alicia to the pediatric oncology unit. She was doing very well, so there was no reason to send her to the Pediatric ICU first. She continued pulling on her tubes until most of them were removed. It was great knowing she would be back in her room soon. The nursing staff instructed me to wait for her there.

I called Dick back to tell him where to find us. He was excited about her being out of ICU so quickly and that she didn't have to go to the pediatric ICU. Being in a room was much more comfortable. In a matter of a couple of hours, she arrived.

Alicia slept for most of the rest of the afternoon. I held and rocked her for a while to give her a change in position, and it gave me an excuse to hold her in my arms. I was surprised she did not seem uncomfortable or in pain after all she had been through. But they had given her medicine to stay ahead of any pain she might have, which made sense. Alicia had some juice and a few bites of Jell-O for supper. She was worn out and seemed pretty content to be rocked.

Dick had come to the hospital after work. He was relieved to see her in her own room again, not hooked to machines or monitors. With Alicia sleeping, after a while he went home to spend a little more time with the boys. He also indicated he needed to do some laundry and mow the lawn, staying busy.

Alicia had a pretty good night. The nurses were in and out to check her vitals and give her pain medicine, but she slept comfortably. I tried getting a little extra sleep, but those couches, though better than nothing, are only comfortable for a short time.

The plan now was to let her recover from the surgery, and then she would start another round of chemotherapy. We would continue with the chemotherapy, even if the pathology report indicated the surgeon had been able to remove the entire tumor. The oncologists wanted to make sure there weren't any cells that had gone astray to cause her problems in the future, so the protocol was to continue chemotherapy.

Alicia grew stronger by the day. The improvement in her shakiness was not immediate, but within a few days, we all noticed some signs of improvement. She was a bit steadier. Her left eyelid drooped terribly, almost to the point of being unable to see her eye. I was told they may have bruised some nerve endings during surgery. If the nerves had been bruised, the droopiness in her eye would improve. If the nerves were damaged, her eye would likely stay that way. Thankfully, her eyelid eventually, slowly but surely, improved. However, even today, when she is tired, her eyelid droops.

Her voice was also very deep and raspy, and the doctors gave me the same explanation. If they had bruised vocal cords, her voice would improve. If they were damaged, that may be as good as it would get. I asked if there were any other surprises yet to appear. They didn't think so. As concerned as we were about these things, we were thankful they were able to remove the tumor. We decided if we got to keep her, we could live with the rest. Eventually, her eye and voice improved; it just took time.

We took one day at a time during the recovery process. Each day, there seemed to be some improvement, even if it was small. Some days, I wondered if I was seeing improvement simply because I wanted to.

HOSPITAL LIFE

Sometimes, if we picked her up wrong, she would wince in pain, but she never cried or whined.

When the surgeons and oncologists decided Alicia was strong enough to start chemo again, we did. I felt so bad for her. I knew she would get violently ill, and with her tender incision and stitches, it seemed it would be very hard on her. I wanted them to give her a few more days to heal, but they were convinced she could handle the chemo, and I had to assume they wouldn't harm Alicia. She, of course, weathered it like a trooper when we started again.

It was, however, a vicious cycle of eating and puking. If we let her have breakfast and then started her chemo, we would get it right back. But it made some sense to try to get calories into her. Either way, she was going to get sick. Each time, when she was through being sick and had a nap, she'd want to hit the halls moving, not returning until meals and/or bedtime. It was tough, but I got pretty good at pushing two IV poles and a stroller with Alicia in it. That may not sound like much of an accomplishment, but those IV tubes like to get tangled around the stroller's wheels! She was content as long as we were on the move, visiting or strolling.

After what seemed like another very long hospital stay, we were finally able to check out and head home. By this time, we'd spent the better part of three weeks each in July, August, and September in the hospital. Somehow, with the help of family and friends, we had managed to get the boys back into school and were moving forward.

I remember getting my paycheck for the month of August. By the time I paid our insurance and other deductions, my take-home pay was seven dollars. Seven dollars is hardly enough to survive on. I'm not sure that even covered a day of parking in the hospital parking ramp. But, of course, that wasn't my priority.

IV
THE NEW NORMAL

The next few months were just days and weeks of roller coaster rides. Alicia continued to improve and gain strength. Some days were better than others, but most of them were moving in a positive direction. We would go into the hospital for five days of chemo, home for two weeks, and then in for five more days of treatment. We held that schedule for two years. There were a few bumps in the road and delays in treatment because her blood counts were low, or the like, but for the most part, that was the schedule the entire family was on for the next two years. Five days in, two weeks at home, five days in... That meant a lot of moving around for the boys. During the summer, especially once swimming lessons and park recreation had wrapped up, we tried to get them somewhere they could play and try to forget some of the problems at home. Once school started, their movement would be limited, so we arranged summer visits with grandparents, aunts, uncles, cousins, and friends as best we could. We needed them to have some sense of normalcy in their lives. As I have said, I can't imagine what we would have done without the help, love, and support of our entire families.

Those two years were certainly days of ups and downs. Fortunately, we had more ups than downs. Generally, improvements were constant. It was amazing how exciting Alicia's "firsts" were to us this time around. We were ecstatic when she could hold a spoon again and feed herself! When she started walking again, using a stroller for support, Vicki suggested we put her accomplishment in the headlines of the local paper. Those "second time" firsts were amazing.

Coping

Coping as a parent gave me a whole new perspective on stress. The possibility of losing your child is overwhelming. Then you throw in the "what did I do to her," and "how could this happen," and the "what ifs," and you can lose your mind trying to make sense of it all. Your mind never shuts down. You never stop thinking about everything around and ahead of you. You can't, or you'll never feel like you're making the right decision. Not only were there decisions to make regarding Alicia's treatment, surgery, and protocol, but we still had two boys at home who needed us as well. As a parent, you worry about your child, the patient. But you also worry about your other children, your parents, and each other, to say nothing of trying to balance jobs and home life, giving the latter some form of normalcy — whatever that might be!

Parents must remember some basic things. No one is the "perfect" parent. You do the best you can with any given circumstance and cannot beat yourself up about decisions you make, even if you are unsure whether the decision was correct down the road. Do the best you can.

Advocate

It took a fair amount of time, but I finally learned you must firmly believe in being your child's advocate and make sure you ask questions. It took quite some time to think I could question the medical professionals. You can. You should. Most health professionals will explain what you are dealing with and help you understand it. A few dislike being questioned, but I never questioned anyone's medical advice or knowledge. I just needed to know why a particular decision was being made. I needed to understand what they were talking about. I had questions that needed answers. How can you expect to make intelligent, well-educated decisions down the road if you don't gather facts and information along the way? You may not use the information you learn today, but I guarantee that at some point in the future, you will use the knowledge you acquired along the way. When your children's lives are at stake, how can parents be expected to accept what the doctors say without asking questions? I think doctors just forget to communicate with parents on a level they can understand. So, it is up to parents to ask questions and protect their children.

Normalcy at home

I don't know if any of us know what normalcy at home really means, but I think of it as getting back into whatever routine a family had before the word "cancer" affected their lives so drastically. For us, it was just having the boys back at home, eating together, spending time together, working together. Aside from financial limitations, we could not get away much or vacation because we needed to avoid exposing Alicia to diseases and the problems they posed for her as a chemo patient. Because Alicia's blood counts were often low and her immune system was compromised, we were trying to keep her from catching anything that would delay her treatment. Dick and I worked when we were not in the hospital with Alicia. Besides our jobs, there were the typical chores, such as housework, laundry, yard work and so on, that needed to be taken care of. Nonetheless, because our time with them was so limited, we made the most of it and spent as much time with the boys as possible. I'm sure they felt like all we ever did was work at home to catch up and try to get ahead with chores. They were probably right.

The stresses and emotions connected to a diagnosis like this are tremendous. And while it was sometimes difficult to accept help from everyone, we had to. Sometimes, the situation was so overwhelming that we just wanted to be alone at home. Sometimes we just needed time to cry privately or spend time with our kids as a family. We had yet to determine how much family time we might be granted. I often think about the fun we missed out on while worrying about her future when Alicia was at that wonderful toddler age. Dick, of course, had a family history he couldn't get out of his mind. Losing his dad at such a young age, he felt he missed out on parts of being a kid and just having his dad in his life. His mom had to pick up the pieces after his dad died. That included finding a job and holding life together for Dick and his five siblings. How much time would we be granted with Alicia?

We also discovered fathers generally don't handle hospitals and illnesses as well as mothers do. Dads are supposed to be able to fix everything. Dads are supposed to be the provider, protector, and strong male figure who makes everything all right. Well, sometimes all of this just isn't possible, and it is difficult for dads to come to terms with that. It is a situation out of their control, and they don't like it. Mothers tend to continue the nurturing they do so well. While Alicia was in treatment, we saw many fathers leave the hospital in anger with everything and everyone around them. However, we never saw a mom leave her child's bedside, no matter how frustrated or upset or horrible things were. Moms just don't leave their babies behind. Generally, however, after a father had time to blow off steam and regroup, he returned ready to cope with whatever the situation. Men and women deal with these things differently, and I don't think anyone can tell you how you might react to any situation. Again, you do your best and live with your decision. Don't second-guess yourselves. And don't judge others in horrible situations. We all handle things differently. You won't always make the right decision. Make the best one you can! And don't expect your faith, no matter how strong, to get you through every day. I guarantee your faith will waiver more than once.

Extended Family

I felt so sorry for the grandparents and the rest of our family members. Everyone was concerned and wanted desperately to help however they could. I'm sure it is such a helpless feeling most of the time. Sometimes, there wasn't anything they could do. However, when we needed help, we had such wonderful support from everyone. Makes us thankful every day!

V
REALITIES AND FRUSTRATIONS

Hospital life takes on a personality all its own. Oh, people can tell you how things will (or should) progress and offer suggestions. We understood friends, family, and even some hospital personnel were only offering what they believed were correct answers. You know everyone has a way of handling these issues and coping with situations. And it seems that even people who haven't experienced any of this have good ideas. Just ask them. They will be glad to tell you the best way. Helpful hints: NO ONE copes the same. NO ONE has the very same feelings. NO ONE has the very same set of problems and protocol. NO ONE has all the right answers. NO ONE can. Not if they are human.

Not all bumps in our lives were created by hospital problems. Dick and I hit a real rough patch in February. It became apparent, according to him, that nothing I ever did at the hospital was right. I didn't ask the right questions; I didn't insist on things happening more quickly. I was the one spending almost every day at the hospital, calling him with whatever the circumstances were, but it was never quite right. It was about the time of them placing Alicia's central line. Looking back, I think it was when nerves were shot and tempers short. Everyone was tired. However, that wasn't my fault. When he came to the hospital this particular night, I met him at the door and told him that if this was what he thought, he could pack his bags and find a new place to live. I'd meet him at the courthouse when Alicia was released from this round of chemotherapy. I didn't have the stamina to fight for Alicia's life and fight him. We left the hospital long enough to grab sandwiches to celebrate Valentine's Day. He didn't pack, and I'm so thankful I didn't have to move on alone, but I think he got the point!

I hesitate to discuss some of the problems we ran into because, at this point, those problems seem minimal and unimportant. We made it through treatment and thank God we have Alicia. However, when we were in the middle of that whirlwind, it was important, frustrating, and irritating. In these 40 years since diagnosis, I have never questioned the expertise and amazing knowledge we experienced and received. On more than one occasion, however, I questioned whether there would have been, and could be, better organization and communication if the health professionals stopped and listened to parents. I understand these sick children are everyone's priority, but sometimes parents may know better about what a child needs, not of a medical nature, but in terms of schedules and comfort. Tests and chemotherapy schedules could be improved if medical staff listened to parents. Perhaps, today, they do, and things run more smoothly, with no irritating glitches for parents and children. I realize medical professionals may not always agree with parents' suggestions. There were often valid reasons why we ran into so many delays. Still, for parents in the middle of this horrific experience, with the possibility of losing their child, the lack of communication and disorganization that sometimes exists seems to be something they should NOT have to deal with. Some of these issues could be avoided, making them one less thing to add to parents' stress levels. All that said, I know we received the best possible care and treatment, and I admire the hematology-oncology doctors and nurses. No one should have to deal with

REALITIES AND FRUSTRATIONS

dying children daily; very few can. It takes an amazingly special breed to care for these children and cope as they do. We have the utmost respect for these professionals who give of their lives as they do and still go home to their own families at night. Surely, they think about the what ifs with their own families.

I hope some of the frustrating issues we encountered have ironed themselves out by now. I am going to believe that they have.

Some of our most frustrating days were spent in the clinics and waiting for tests. We discussed this frustration in support group meetings. Several participant parents and one of the top orthopedic doctors at UIHC, whose daughter had cancer, agreed the pediatric clinic was one of the biggest offenders for management of time issues. Everyone understands how appointments and tests can get off schedule but running that way continuously seems uncalled for and a major problem when dealing with sick children and their families. These families are already dealing with illnesses beyond their control. I believe an advocate or advocacy group would help communication between stressed parents and medical staff.

Alicia spiked a temperature one of the very first evenings in the hospital. After paging the on-call doctors and engaging in much discussion, the decision was made for her to undergo an X-ray. However, for some reason, we were sent to the part of the hospital that performed CAT scans. One of the staff just handed Alicia to me and said, "Go here, go there, and then up the ramp, and don't be confused because at the end of the ramp, you hit a different number floor. The new part of the hospital is numbered differently than the old part of the hospital, and here are her charts. We'll see you when you return from there." Not being accustomed to the system, I took Alicia, and away I went. Now I'm about halfway to the scanner. I think, "What the hell am I doing out here?!" It is now midnight, I'm wandering around a hospital I don't know anything about with a toddler with a life-threatening illness, and I don't know where the hell I am. I continued to get increasingly disgusted with the floor staff for sending me out on my own and mad at God because my child was sick. The madder I got, the faster I walked, and the closer I got to tears. I kept wondering how I let this happen. Why didn't I tell them I didn't know where I was going? Why didn't I ask someone to go along with me? Why didn't I ask some questions? Funny how we learn some things the hard way. Eventually, we got the test done, and I started wandering back with my baby. Even though Alicia was little, she got pretty heavy by the time we got from one end of the hospital to the other. It was about 2 a.m. when we got back to her room. I never made a trip like that again alone.

In another instance, Alicia had a CAT scan scheduled for mid-afternoon. I think this was when they were looking for tumors in her brain and possibly on her eyes. The sedation process was started, and Alicia was prepped for the scan. About the time she was due in the CAT scan clinic, there was an emergency, and she was bumped from the schedule. Everyone understands an emergency; I'd hope someone else would understand if it were my emergency. Okay, a little more sedation was needed because the original dose would have worn off before the scan was completed. After a while, we were told that one of the scanners had broken down, the other one was backed up, and they were attempting to get a portable scanner to help with the situation. More sedation was needed to keep her sleeping because we could still get the scan in that night. At about 7 p.m., we were notified that a portable scanner was downstairs just off the emergency room entrance, and that they could take Alicia there for her scan. So, downstairs we go with our sleeping baby girl in a tin cart. They put us in a little waiting room, taking Alicia outside to the portable scanner.

The equipment appeared to be in a semi-trailer parked in the parking lot next to the emergency room. At least, that's where they took our little girl. It wasn't high-tech and certainly not very comforting to see, but we hoped to get the scan done. By this time, everyone, including the housekeeping personnel, had left for the day. I didn't know where to find any staff; I didn't know exactly where my child was . . . hell, I didn't know if we were locked in or out! But we sat and waited patiently, assuming

REALITIES AND FRUSTRATIONS

someone would come back with Alicia or tell us what to do next. Someone came about 8 p.m. to tell us that this portable machine had now stopped functioning, and we would have to take her to the other end of the hospital again (where I went in the middle of the night) to finish her scans. In the meantime, someone from our floor was coming to give Alicia a little more sedation. Away we went with our sleeping girl in the tin tub. We waited patiently for them to finish a scan they were in the middle of, only to be told that the portable scanner was back up and running, and they'd really prefer to finish Alicia's scans on that one since it was where they started. SO, back down to the first floor to the parking lot by the emergency entrance we went. The scan was finally completed, and we got back to the second floor at about 10 p.m. (Hospital personnel were always amazed when parents lost their tempers. Imagine.) So, we settled in for the night. Alicia had enough sedation to sleep through the night, oblivious to what had transpired. There were things to be thankful for.

And then there was the time we had to come in for a scan when the only opening was very early in the morning. It was scheduled for something like 7 or 7:30 a.m. Due to insurance regulations, we were unable to be inpatients the night before. We had to come from Tipton early in the morning for the prep work. We made arrangements at home with the boys and left at 4 a.m. When we reached the hospital, we had to go to the floor for prepping because the clinic was not open yet. Whoever had to write the orders for the gook Alicia had to drink before the scan had not written them, and the night shift staff could not write the orders. No one in the pharmacy could send the stuff she needed to drink until they had written orders. So, we sat and we waited for several hours, and then, when the orders were written and the gook arrived, a nurse informed us we only had 30 minutes to get this 2-year-old to drink a god-awful amount of ill-tasting mixture so we could get her to the scanner and stay on schedule. I think she knew from the looks she got from both Dick and me that that wasn't going to happen, and someone had better make the necessary change in scheduling. We had to wait a while to be worked in, but we got the scan done that morning, lucky for everyone connected to that boo boo.

It seemed we always had to be on top of things. At one point, after we were well into treatment, the doctors wanted to decrease the dosage of one of the chemo drugs. Blood was discovered in Alicia's urine, and they indicated one of the drugs could cause that, but by cutting back, we'd be OK. When the script came to the floor with the same dosage, I had to argue with one of the interns about giving her that dose. I can't imagine what patients who don't have a support system do, or what happens to patients with a family that doesn't pay attention.

Another day, when I was sitting with Alicia waiting for a scan, an elderly man was sitting in his wheelchair, sleeping. He was there when we arrived and still there when we left. I was afraid he was going to fall out of his chair. Dick wondered if someone had forgotten him there or if he'd been there all night. Sometimes we wondered, especially if a patient didn't have a spokesperson.

I had decided to work one day when my mom and dad were going to be at the hospital, and nothing much was going on. Late in the morning, hospital staff came to Alicia's room to get her for surgery. Thank God my mother was there. Alicia was not scheduled for any kind of surgery. Just imagine someone getting between a grandmother and her granddaughter. It wasn't going to happen.

Some glitches were not always hospital related. Sometimes it was the insurance companies. We shared hospital life with a farm family from northwest Iowa. Their son was also fighting neuroblastoma; his tumor was in his abdomen. Their drill was similar to ours, with a number of days in and then so many days at home. For most of his protocol, they would come down to the UIHC the day before they started treatment to do X-rays and blood work. Then the next morning, they were ready to start his chemo. This particular time, Dad dropped Mom and their son off at the door and headed back home. I don't remember whether it was planting or harvesting season, but Dad went home to return to the field. In trying to get admitted, they learned their insurance company would no longer cover the cost of staying overnight, and they'd have to go home and return the next morning. Since this was before everyone had a cell phone, Mom and Derek had to sit and wait for Dad to get home, call him, and then wait for him to get back to Iowa City. This had to be an 8-to-10-hour process. What do you do with a young child for 8-10 hours in a hospital setting? I imagine that when Dad returned to Iowa City, they just got a motel room for the night. Nothing was ever easy for families already struggling.

There was the time when we had been in the hospital for chemo and then home for a few days, and Alicia spiked a temperature. Because temperatures, low blood counts, and chemo can cause horrible problems, we were instructed to bring Alicia into the emergency room at UIHC since the clinic was closed. We arrived around 6:30 p.m., waited to be seen in the emergency department, and then waited for hospital personnel to order bloodwork sent to the lab "STAT." We waited until 2 a.m. for those results and for the doctors to admit Alicia to the hospital. I'd hate to think how long results take if they are sent "non-STAT." Dick went home to be with the boys, and I stayed with Alicia.

We got to the hematology/oncology floor sometime after 3 a.m. and had just settled in for a little sleep when I heard furniture moving and doors banging. So I looked out in the hallway. There was a child a couple of doors down who had broken out with chickenpox. Chickenpox and chemotherapy can prove fatal, so they were moving the child and sanitizing the room. Things weren't always easy for staff either!

Alicia had several bone marrow tests, keeping an eye out for whether the cancer was spreading into her marrow. Anyone who has been down this path knows that retrieving bone marrow is extremely painful. They drew marrow from both sides of her lower back, causing it to be painful for her to walk for a few days. She'd have large bandages on both little butt cheeks below her waist. Once she endured all this only to discover there had been an error SOMEWHERE BY SOMEONE with her marrow, and they would need to draw again. We never received an explanation of whether it was lost, damaged, or what. I wasn't happy with that one.

Along with all these "situations," others stand out as being the most frustrating of our treatment time. The first one was a day when Alicia was again scheduled for a CAT scan and to be seen in Nuclear Medicine. We had to be in the clinic early in the morning, which suited us best, in hopes schedules weren't already running behind. We started in the clinic at 8 a.m. with routine check-in and blood work. Soon to follow was getting an IV started and then sedation. It was about time to go to the CAT scanner when we got word that an emergency would delay Alicia's scan. OK, we understood delays. Alicia was given more sedation at about 10 a.m. because we would be next in line for a scan. Soon after 10 a.m., we were sent to CAT scan at the opposite end of the hospital. We sat, and we waited, and we waited. At about noon, someone from our floor administered additional sedation to Alicia. She was still sleeping in her tin tub, but we knew she'd never make it through the entire scan without waking up, and she wouldn't lie still without the sedation. At 12:45 p.m., I went up to the desk to inform the woman sitting there that we were due for a bone scan in Nuclear Medicine at 1 p.m. I told her we would go to Nuclear Medicine and be back for the CAT scan. She snarled at me that they were about ready to take Alicia in, and I couldn't take her from the area. I explained to her that we had been on the schedule at 8 a.m. and had been bumped and delayed, and now, I was taking her to Nuclear Medicine for the bone scan, and then we would be back. As I pushed the tin tub with my sleeping baby down the hall, the attendant informed me that if I took her from the area, I would give up any right to get Alicia's CAT scan, which would be rescheduled for another day. I was proud of myself this time. I didn't even get angry. I spun around on my heels, walked back to her desk, and quietly and calmly informed her that we had an appointment at 1 p.m. in Nuclear Medicine, where I was going with Alicia. I also told her we would be back and that I would expect them to find a slot for Alicia's scan before day's end. We weren't the problem. We had been there all morning waiting patiently and letting them give her more and more sedation. We would run the scan before anyone left for the day. She just sat and stared at me, like how dare I speak to her that way. And then I added with a smile, "If this is how you want to treat human beings, you really should be putting labels on cans at H.J. Heinz instead of harassing the human race and people who needed some compassion." I turned and walked away. On the way to Nuclear Medicine, I walked right past the head of the CAT scan department and invited myself into his office. I calmly told him of my experience and the day's activities, and that now we were going to keep our appointment in Nuclear Medicine. I would be back, and I expected a slot for Alicia before the end of the day. As soon as we had completed the bone scan, I took my little girl in her tin tub back to the CAT scan area, smiled at the commandant behind the desk, and sat down. Amazingly enough, we only waited for about an hour, and there was an opening for Alicia.

The second major frustration was after we reached a point in Alicia's protocol to do the first couple of days of her chemo in the hospital because she had to be hydrated, and then the next several days could be done at home. We had been doing this regimen for several months. We would go in on Thursday afternoon and do blood work, exam, and chest X-rays if the hematology-oncology doctors thought any were necessary. Alicia was hooked up to hydration so that she could have her first drugs on Friday morning. Saturday, she'd get the second round and then Sunday morning, her third treatment. If everything had gone well, we could check out and go home. We were only in the hospital for a few days and home again, which seemed to work well. Sunday morning, at 10 a.m., all was well. I packed her up, and we were about ready to leave the hospital. It would be so good to get back home to the boys. During this series of treatments, Dick was usually at home with the boys.

I had my toddler and all our belongings in the hallway when an intern informed me that they needed a chest X-ráy.

"For what?" I asked.

"It's routine," he told me.

"It can't be too routine. We have never done one on Sunday morning before going home."

"Well, we should have. It's routine," was his retort.

I persisted, "Well, we haven't, so I don't see any reason to do one now." I asked him if they were looking for something with the chest X-ray.

"No, it's just routine," he said.

"Then, as her mom, I can't justify putting her through more X-rays just because you tell me it's routine."

He insisted they would do the X-ray before we were allowed to leave.

"Really? Well, you get me Dr. Raymond Tannous (he was the staff physician on call) on the phone, and if he can give me a good reason as to why we NEED to have an X-ray, then we'll have an X-ray. Short of that, we aren't going to."

After the intern called Dr. Tannous and explained what was going on, I spoke with Dr. Tannous, who informed me there was no reason to have the X-ray, as they weren't looking for anything specific. If he thought there were any problems, we would have done the X-ray when we were admitted on Thursday. So, it was certainly up to me. When I got off the phone, the intern again told me we had to do the chest X-ray, or he wouldn't sign off on our release papers. I picked up my toddler and our belongings and told him I was going home to my family. He had my home address, and if he chose to send my release papers to me, my address was in Alicia's charts. If he chose not to, I didn't much care where he stuck them. We never received our release papers from that visit.

REALITIES AND FRUSTRATIONS

I picked up our hospital STUFF and took my daughter by the hand. We were heading home. We got to the elevator, Alicia pushed the down button, the doors opened, I put our suitcases inside and I turned to pick up a second load of belongings. Alicia got in the elevator. The doors closed with her in the elevator and me on the outside. Panic. Where would the doors open and she might step out? Would someone find her and kidnap her? Would someone find her and take her to security? Should I start down the stairwell? Should I call security? LOTS of thoughts can go through your mind in short order! Before I could decide and make any move, the doors opened, and there stood my brown-eyed girl.

Due to the length of Alicia's protocol and the number of chemo treatments, a central line was surgically placed in her chest when we were about six months into treatment. This alleviates the constant poking and starting IVs for blood draws and chemotherapy administration. We waited the six months because central lines are prone to infection in approximately a year and we still had about two years ahead of us. This meant I had to learn how to flush the central line daily and take care of it so infection did not start. We were BLESSED with good luck and no infection.

The third incident occurred when we were preparing to remove Alicia's central line at the end of her treatment. We were scheduled to be at the surgical clinic at 1 p.m. We arrived on time, and at about 2 p.m., I asked if they knew how much longer we would have to wait. We needed to sedate Alicia for this procedure, pull her central line, and let her have time to recover. This is not a clinic that is open after 5 p.m. I was told, "A while." I asked what "a while" meant. The answer was, "A while." When asked whether there was any idea if "a while" is 20 minutes or 2 hours, the response was no, they didn't know, but I should take a seat. It would still be "a while." We were told one of the doctors was in Australia, and they were behind schedule. With that, absolutely furious, I left Alicia with my parents and stormed (literally) into the office of one of the top UIHC administrators, who was also our neighbor in Tipton. I was livid. I was tired and frustrated and probably past making much sense, but I intended to make someone notice people are tired of waiting and never getting a straight answer. He calmed me down. I'm not sure he said much; I was doing all the talking. But he offered me a chair, listened to me expound on my experience yet again, and then picked up the phone. He was going to call the clinic to see if he could find out what was happening and how long "a while" might be. They offered him the same song and dance about one of the doctors being on vacation and not telling him the length of "a while," and he became fairly short with them, indicating they needed to find out what "a while" meant so they could inform patients who were waiting. We visited a little longer, and he, of course, asked about Alicia. By the time I left his office, I felt better. Not that I wasn't still tired of the run around, but he was calming. I wasn't back in the clinic for more than 15 minutes when Alicia's name was called. They put us into one of the little rooms to wait for the doctor. Within another 15 or 20 minutes, the doctor, who was supposedly in Australia, walked through our door. When I questioned how his vacation was and whether he had just arrived from the airport, he looked at me, extremely confused. I told him the story the reception staff fed me and the administrator. He was not happy. I assume nothing more came of that, but I did return and let the administrator know he had been lied to. And yes, ultimately, we did get Alicia's central line pulled and made our way out of the clinic. It was just another one of those things that didn't need to happen.

Not ALL bad

With what sounds like a fair amount of complaining, we also had some good times and found things to laugh about. Sometimes Ladonna and I would laugh over nothing at all, or we'd start out crying about something and end up laughing. We were often in the hospital together for treatment, and those visits seemed more manageable. One day, Ladonna made strawberry daiquiris and put them in a cooler to bring to the hospital. When the kids were all tucked in for the night, we sat in our shared bathroom on the floor, leaning against the bathtub, and drank strawberry daiquiris. We've laughed about that night numerous times. One of our favorite interns caught us, but he didn't tell the authorities. He must have known we needed that.

There was also the time my brother Tom called to say he was coming to Iowa City. Did I need anything? I said, "YES! I need a beer." After Alicia was settled in for the night, Tom and I went out to his van, and I sat and drank a beer or two. I went back into the hospital with a whole new perspective. Sometimes I just needed to get out of there and regroup. On that occasion, my optimism had much more to do with the change of scenery and the company than the beer.

One of my favorite positive memories was when Alicia was at her worst with the shakiness and smeared orange Popsicle all over Dr. Tannous's white coat while we were standing in the hall talking to him. He just grinned at me and said, "Don't worry. . . you're paying to have it cleaned." Dr. Tannous is a very gentle man with a wonderful sense of humor, and to this day, I enjoy visiting with him. Children who survive must be a real emotional lift for medical professionals.

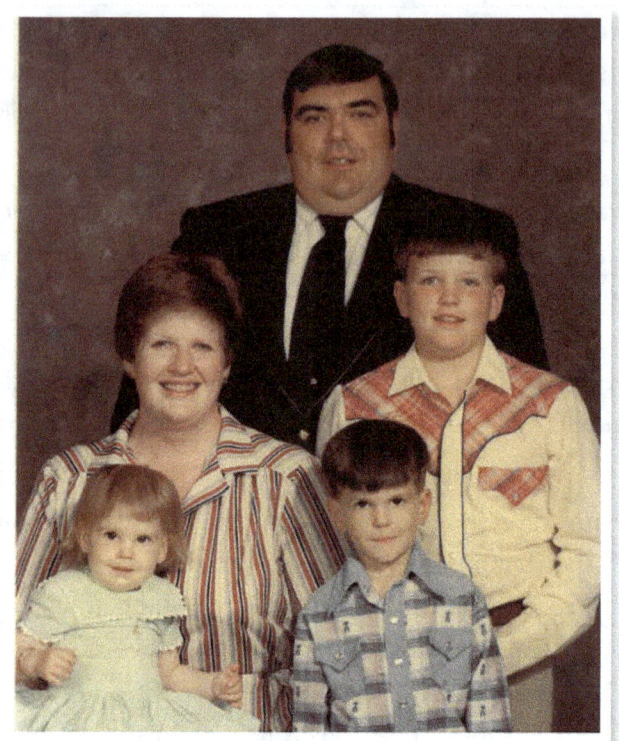
Timm family_1980s

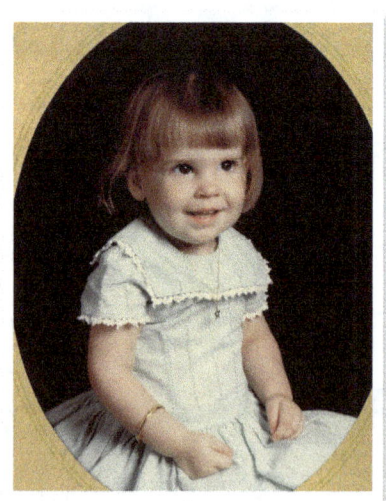
Alicia

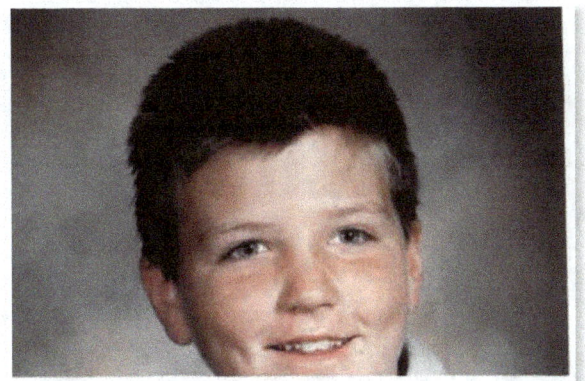
Tony

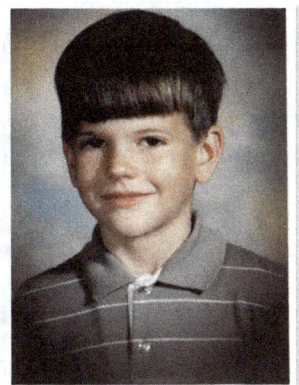
Andy

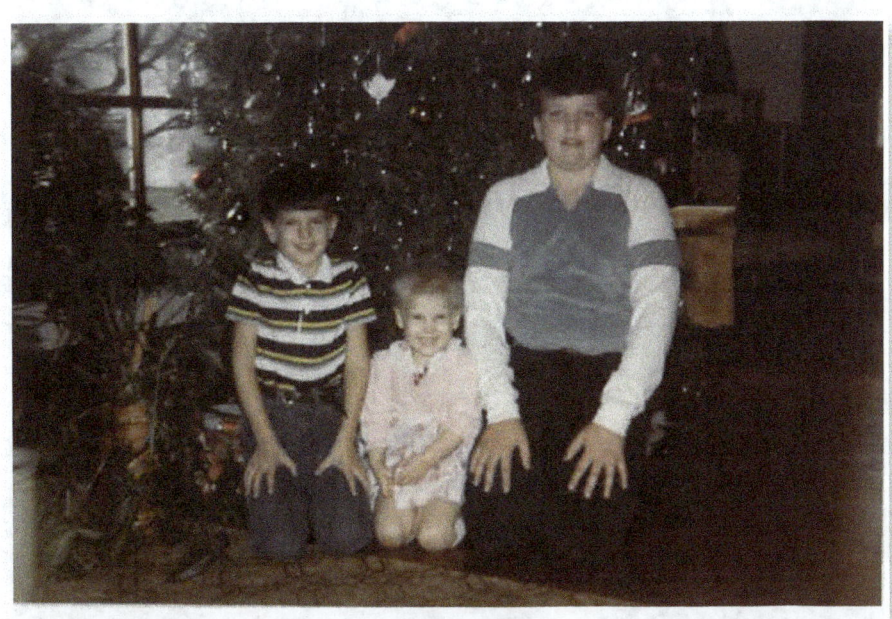
Timm siblings

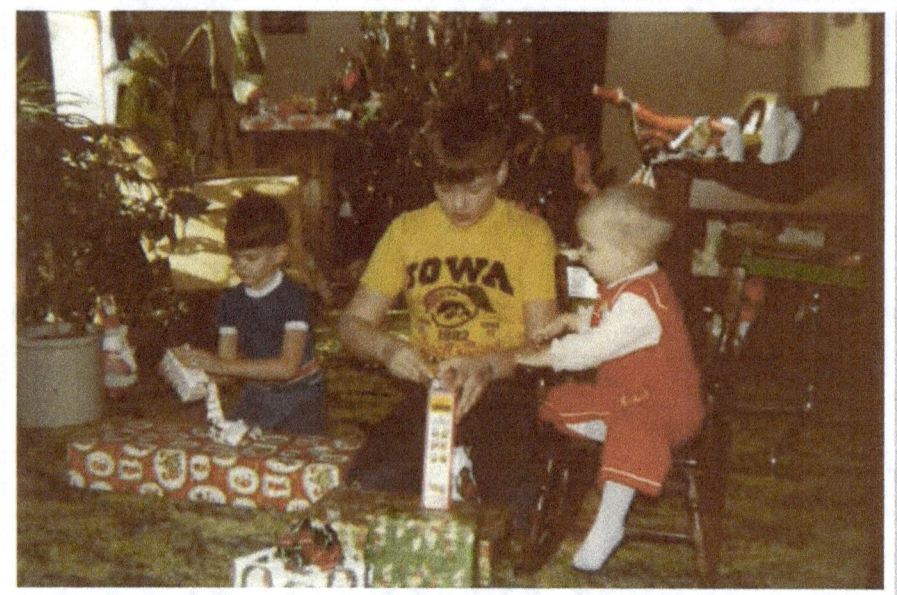
Christmas

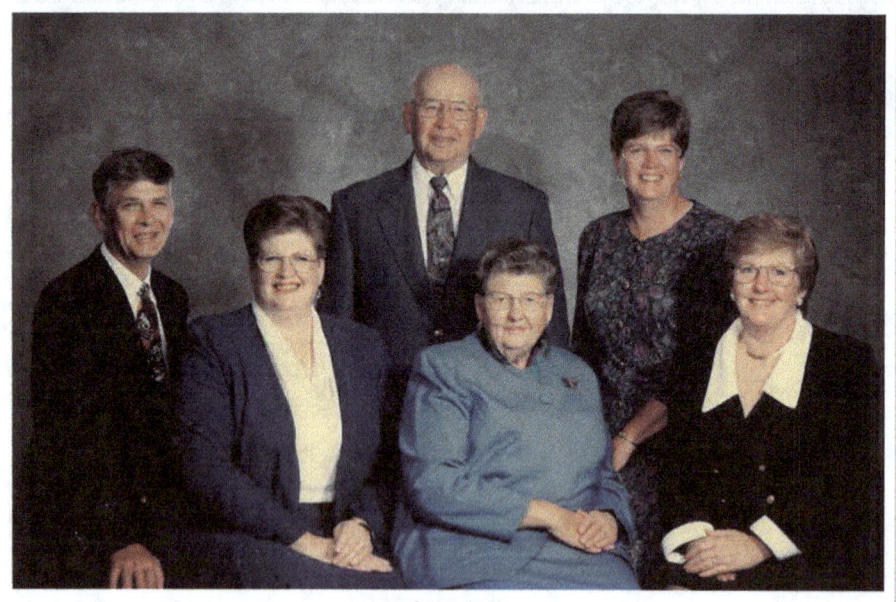
Lilienthals

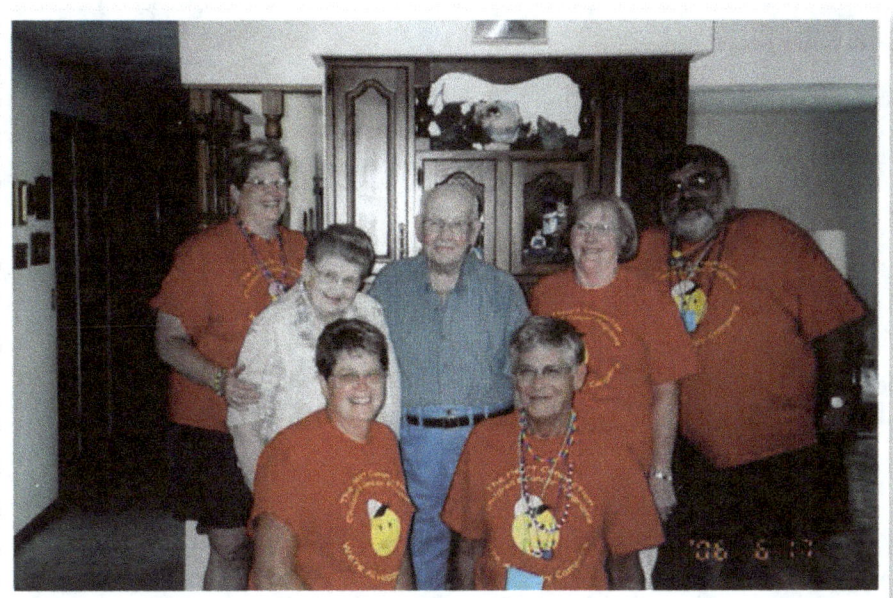
Lillienthals and Dick

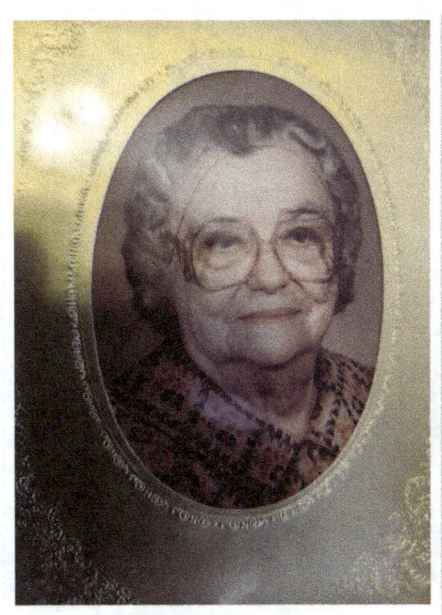
Grandma Timm

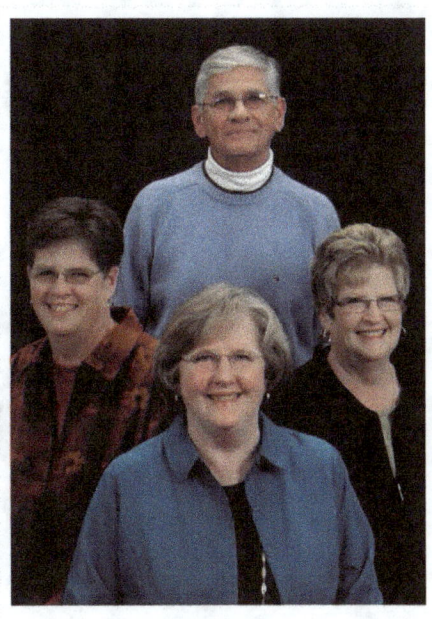
Peggy Sibs

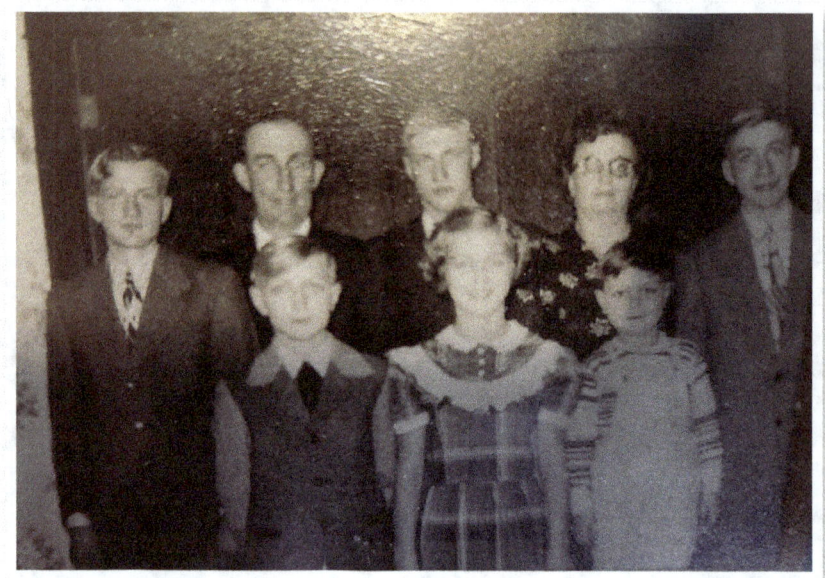

Grandma and Grandpa Timm with Dick and 5 siblings

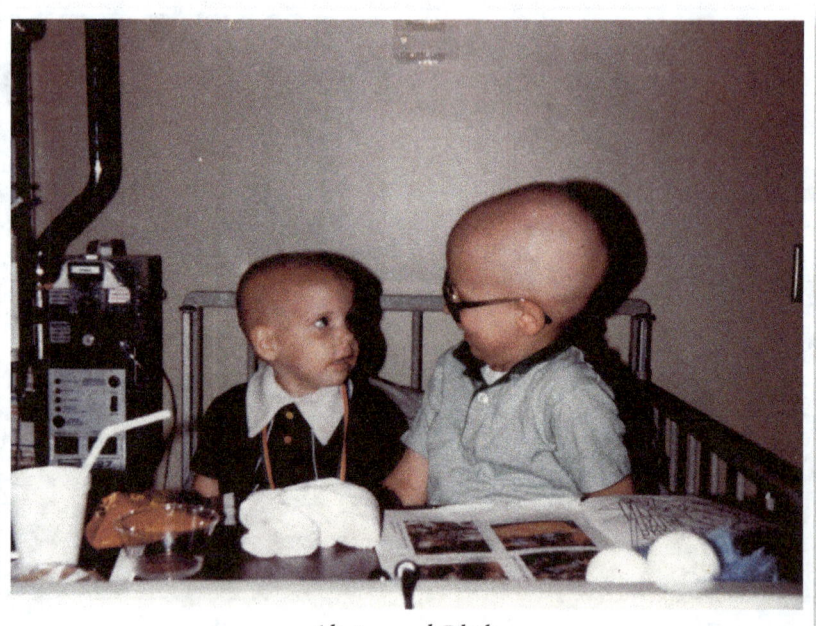

Alicia and Philip

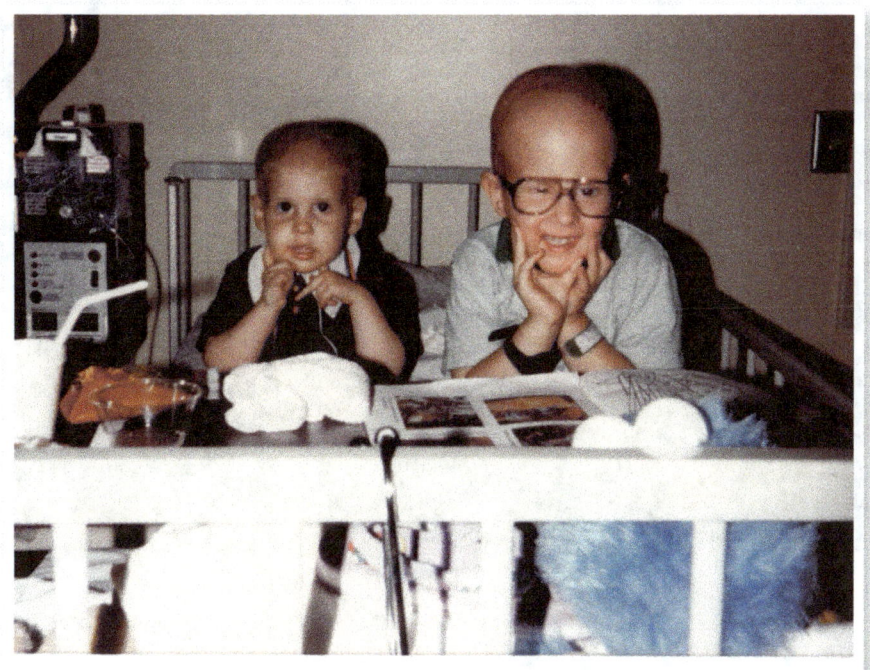

Alicia and Philip

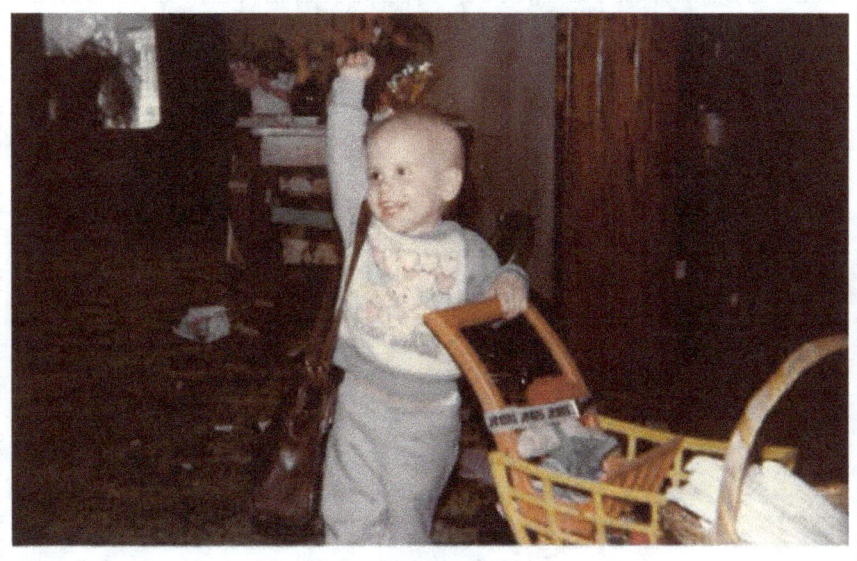

Alicia (relearning to walk)

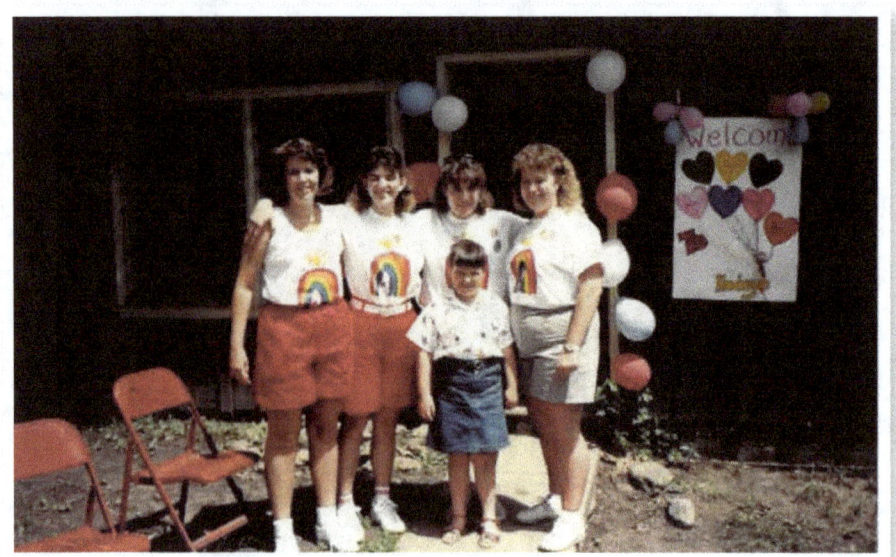

Camp

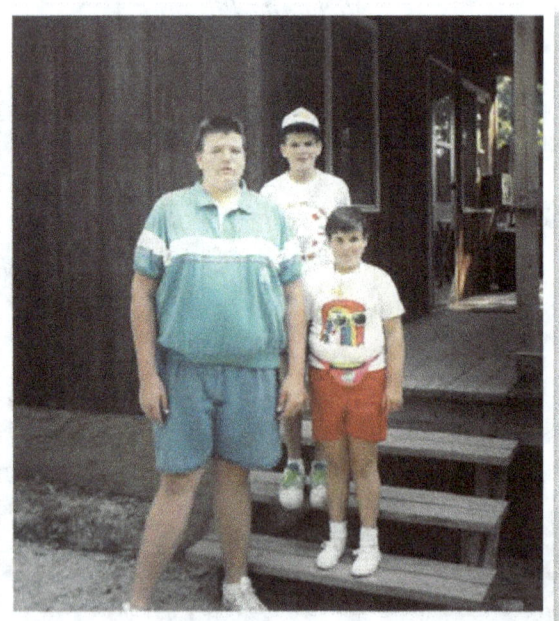

Timm siblings camp

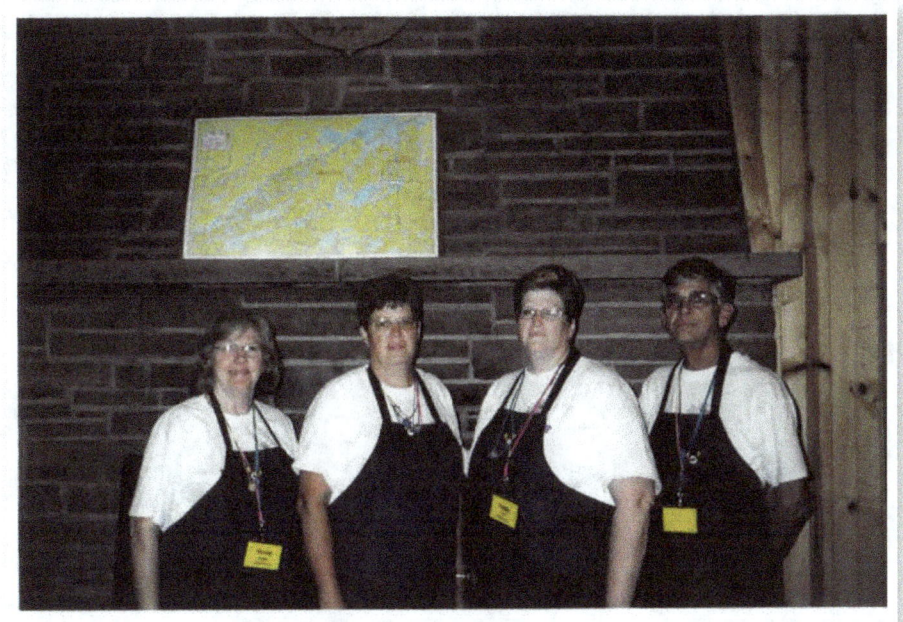

Peggy and siblings at camp

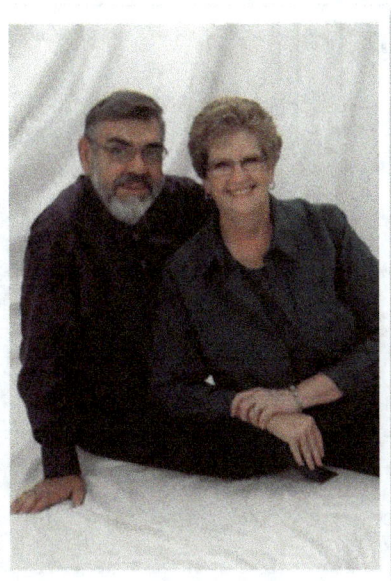

Dick & Peggy

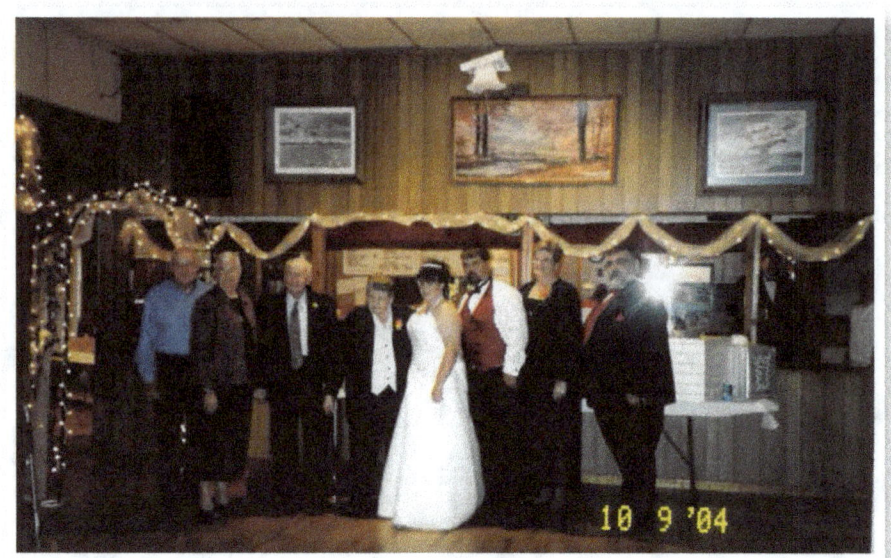

Alicia's wedding

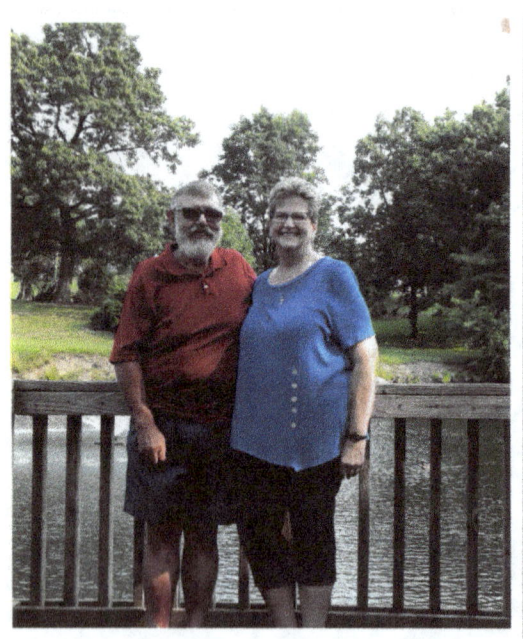

Dick & Peggy

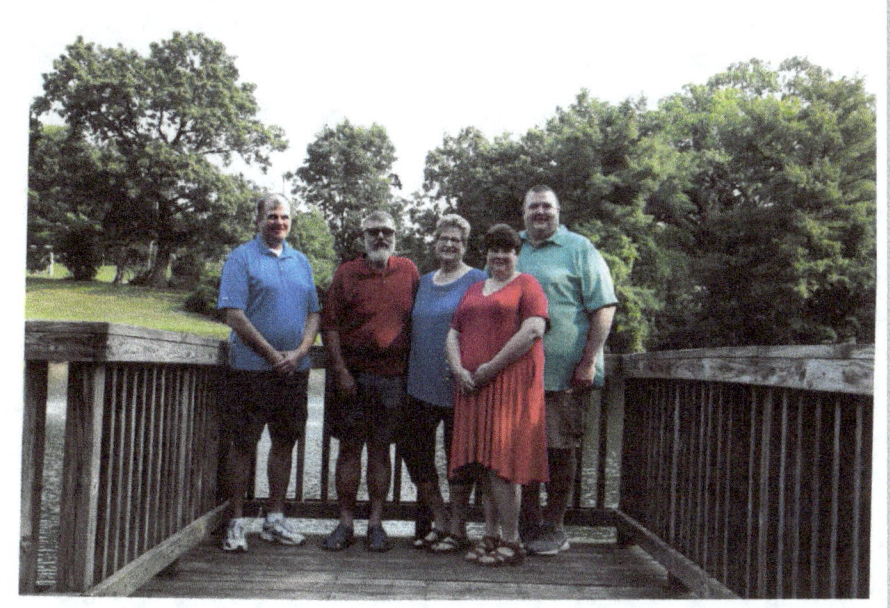
Timm family

VI
SIBLINGS

The amount of information you need to absorb in a short amount of time during the diagnosis stage is incomprehensible. One of the healthcare professionals said, "Cancer is a disease that affects the entire family." Initially, I gave little thought to this statement. There were so many other decisions to be made and obstacles to overcome, but it didn't take long to realize this diagnosis would take over the lives of our entire family for the next two-plus years. We would be at the mercy of health care professionals, schedules, tests, blood counts, and Alicia's reactions to the chemotherapy for a long time. This was one of the times — there were many — when I had to remember to take one day at a time. Sometimes, it was half days at a time; Dick and I believe we did the best we could to keep life moving in a forward direction.

As parents, I don't think you can ever second guess yourselves. I don't know if our boys would necessarily agree, but for the most part, I think they have weathered Alicia's illness with grace. They are wonderful, strong, independent young men. We are an extremely close family. I want to think we would have been anyhow because of our relationships with our children and family values, but I don't know that. I have never doubted Alicia's illness has probably brought us even closer as a family than we might have been. We certainly never take anything for granted and appreciate each and every day God grants us. Many, many families are not as lucky as we are.

Nonetheless, I have sometimes wondered if the boys thought it was unfair that Alicia was getting all the attention. People brought gifts to the hospital or stopped at the house with a little something for her. She was, of course, thrilled. That had to be hard for the boys to see. In fact, the boys occasionally comment about how their sister got everything and how she spent their inheritance, but it is all in fun. At the time, they didn't complain, but I later discovered they were not always the perfect little boys their mom thought they were. And although they claim to have been scarred for life when Aunt Vicki made them eat lima beans during one of their stays at the Meyers's home, they have forgiven her. They still like to kid her, but they have forgiven her.

Tony often refers to this period as being "shipped off" to family and friends. I guess, in all honesty, that is at least partially true. We didn't have a lot of choices when we needed to be in the hospital for treatment. Dick or I had to work. Tony and Andy could not stay at home alone, and we never knew whether our hospital stay would be extended from one day to the next. Everything seemed to be out of our hands, out of our control.

Now, in my defense, we always "shipped" the boys off to somewhere where they would get plenty of love and attention. Grandma and Grandpa Lilienthal, Grandma Timm, or aunts and uncles. There were even a few times when we imposed on friends to keep them for a few days. I think the boys would be the first to admit they were always well cared for.

I am sure this was toughest on Tony because of his age. He had a much stronger understanding of how sick his sister was. He was old enough to know that many people did not survive cancer. We had lost a very dear friend, a grandfather figure to our kids, not long before Alicia's diagnosis. We had lost Vonnie's husband, Loren, to cancer, and although Tony was not old enough to remember a lot about Loren, he knew Loren was not among the fortunate few to survive.

Tony admits to not really knowing what he was feeling, much less understanding his feelings. At first, being moved around was kind of fun. They didn't have to do chores at home and always had somewhere new to play. Going with Aunt Mary to the bakery before school was great because they got to eat donuts. Riding the four-wheeler at Oscar and Vicki's, playing in the hog building and shooting sparrows with BB guns at Harold and Sharon's, playing in the giant room at Vonnie's, playing in the giant yard at Tom and Sally's, sleeping on Grandma Timm's hide-a-bed, eating grilled cheese sandwiches at Nannie's, cracking walnuts in the garage with Ted's clamp and smashing them with his hammer, and riding Grandma and Grandpa's bikes all over Durant were all fun things. However, after a while, the excitement wore off. Riding the school bus to Roger and Mary's, eating lima beans at Vicki's, hearing for the eight millionth time that kids used to be seen and not heard from Grandma Timm, and having to take a nap at Aunt Vonnie's ranked at the top of their not-so-great times with family.

Tony was in the fourth grade when Alicia first entered treatment, and he really struggled in school. Thankfully, Tony's teacher, Mrs. Rosemary Penningroth, had the patience of a saint with him and with us. While in and out of the hospital, I completely lost track of things happening at school. Mrs. Penningroth had to call to see if we could sign and return Tony's report cards. We hadn't even seen Tony's report cards. It seems there was a bit of a fire in Tony's wastebasket one day, and those report cards just happened to be the source of the fire. And it was Tony who built a fire under the porch. He discovered that fingernail polish remover worked pretty well for starting fires, which was an easy way to get rid of unfavorable progress reports.

All was not lost, however. I remember several years later telling Mrs. Penningroth that the kid we thought might be a fourth-grade dropout was on the honor roll in high school.

In addition to issues at school, over the years, Tony has confessed to some of the "naughty" things he did. He "borrowed" my Avon samples to give to the girls in his class so they would like him. He bullied his brother into trips to the grocery store or the Dairy Queen (DQ) using money he had "borrowed" from my purse. Poor Andy was afraid of his big brother and did as he was told. It is also worth noting that you can't live in a town the size of Tipton and not get caught for some of your mischievous deeds. Tony took a silver dollar from a jar of Dick's coins and went to the DQ. The owner of the DQ called to see if we really wanted him to spend the silver dollar, saying that if not, he'd be glad to return it. I admired the DQ owner for going to the trouble and taking the time to contact us. Of course, Tony wasn't happy when we came down on him, and it took him a while to confess, but he did. The boys also confessed to breaking some garage windows when Grandma and Grandpa stayed with them. It wasn't the neighbor boys, after all.

Tony loved seeing if he could get five pieces of Bubblicious Bubble gum in his mouth all at once like the major league baseball players, and he took money from my purse to buy goldfish at the local dime store for his homeroom class at school to enjoy.

We couldn't be at home and with the boys as much as we should have, so these things happened. I don't believe any of it was done to be violent or malicious, but rather to get some attention. We still love you, boys!

On the other hand, Andy just kind of plodded along. I think he did more internalizing than Tony did, but was pretty content to go with the flow and do what needed to be done. He was only 5 years old, and I don't think he understood the severity of his sister's illness like Tony did.

Andy did not start school in the fall when Alicia was diagnosed. He had speech issues, and with us being gone so much, we felt it was better to keep him out of school, get him help with his speech, and let him start the next fall. That was one of the best decisions we made. I don't think he would have done well in school, given everything else going on in his life.

And Andy's claim of mistreatment is that since no one was home to fix them anything to eat, he had to pick up rocks from the alley, and for breakfast, he poured milk over them. They poured hot water over rocks to make soup for lunch and supper. During part of Alicia's chemo at home, she had to drink LARGE amounts of liquids for hydration. When it became difficult for her to drink more water and juices, she ate watermelon. Andrew claims he could never have watermelon because of his little sister. He was, however, permitted to suck the juice off the seeds. He tells people how he was the "Cinderella" of our household. He had to clean the basement and the attic all by himself. He had to scrub the outside of the house and clean the dirt out of the cracks of the sidewalk, all with a toothbrush. These chores, he claims, were all to keep him busy and out of trouble. He also insists that since Alicia has spent her share of their inheritance on hospital and medical bills, she should forgo any inheritance when we are gone. Since it was the boys who suffered, and she got all the toys and attention, they (he and Tony) should be the only ones to inherit anything. THANKFULLY, he doesn't honestly believe any of these things. . . I don't think!

When the boys came to the hospital to see their sister, if they couldn't come to her room for some reason, they stayed in the waiting room. Apparently, Tony snooped through all the cupboards in the waiting room and even tried to get into the locked library book return box. Figuring the padlock was a bit smarter than he was as a 9- or 10-year-old, he finally gave up.

Tony also became tired of being responsible for his little brother. When we were in the hospital, if he wanted to play with friends, Grandma Timm thought he should take his little brother along. He claims he couldn't go anywhere without hearing, "Take your brother, watch your brother, be nice to your brother, share with your brother, give your brother what he wants because he is younger and doesn't understand." I'm sure at his age, his little brother was an annoyance. A cute annoyance (to me), however.

He also remembers some stressful times at home. Like when I took my frustrations out on the door, and the glass in the old door shattered. Or like when his dad threw a Tupperware glass, and it shattered. Tupperware isn't supposed to break . . . much less shatter. Tony admits to being afraid we were one argument away from divorce and that we would make the boys choose where they wanted to live. He is thankful it never happened. Stress and anxiety have to be dealt with, and it may not have been the right way, but, in retrospect, shattered glass and Tupperware were pretty minor.

Thinking back, I'm not sure how we did it. Certainly, we did things wrong or things someone did not approve of, but we did our best. When we were in the hospital with Alicia for treatment, the boys had to be with someone else. When we were at home and Alicia's blood counts were low, we had to ask people not to visit. We couldn't take any chances of her contracting something else to fight.

Just like I don't think anyone can understand what parents or patients go through unless they have been in those shoes, I truly don't believe that anyone can understand what siblings go through. Parents have a whole different set of fears than siblings and grandparents. As parents, we try to protect and explain things as best we can. I guarantee no one does that perfectly. I'm sure the boys had concerns we never addressed and were probably afraid to ask. We've been thankful so many times that Alicia was the age she was. She just thought what she was going through was a part of life. She didn't have to miss school. She didn't have to deal with peers making unkind comments about hair loss and looking "different." Most of all, she never had to understand the severity of her illness and all the "what ifs." She had no idea what could be ahead. However, the boys did.

Tony remembers being called "the boys with the sick sister." We are truly blessed to have survived, all of us!

In general, the boys were real troopers. When I think back, their lives were in turmoil — turmoil they never really understood. Their sister was in and out of the hospital, taking Mom and Dad away from them and taking them away from their home and toys, while Alicia was the one getting more presents and attention.

Despite the broken windows and burned report cards, I am very pleased to say that Tony and Andy made it through the entire ordeal admirably. Just as I believe that no one can understand what a parent with a sick child goes through unless they have had to do it, I also believe we can't possibly comprehend how siblings cope. Being in this situation is not anyone's choice.

Despite everything that happened during that time, I believe the boys have grown into fine, upstanding young men who are very successful in their careers and outstanding husbands and fathers. They have weathered the storm very well. They still love their little sister and are very close to her. Tony admits that truism easier than Andy, but he has clever little ways of letting his sister know she is pretty important to him.

VII

COST OF CARE AND SMALL-TOWN SUPPORT

One thing we learned very quickly is the financial burdens were going to be astronomical. It is unlikely the average person without insurance could stay ahead of the bills that were about to come.

When we started at Mercy, a private hospital room was about $250 per day. When we arrived at the UIHC a few days later, the charge was $500 per day for a semi-private room, and $500 per visit for the staff oncologist, whether or not we ever saw him. Thankfully, we had good insurance because it became apparent there was no way out of this without it.

I remember looking at the hospital bills and being astonished by the charges. A box of diapers was at least four times what they were at the store. We were not allowed, however, to bring diapers with us because of sterility issues. A few feet of new IV tubing was half a week's pay. There were things we (or our insurance company) paid for that I could not believe would be on the bill when we were paying $500 a day for a room. There wasn't much we could do, though; we needed to be there, especially since what we were doing seemed to be working. I can't imagine being a family that incurs that kind of expense and then pays the ultimate price when their child does not survive.

From the time we started at the UIHC in July 1983 until February 1, 1984, Alicia's in-hospital and medical costs hit the $100,000 mark, and then I just stopped counting. The $100,000 included scores of tests, two major surgeries, and chemotherapy. What our insurance did not cover was our responsibility.

Sometimes, I wish I continued to keep track of the costs, but figuring out hospital bills could have become a full-time job. In addition, the bills were difficult to read, and I just didn't have the time or energy to try and figure them out. In the end, I'm not sure we would have wanted to know the final cost of Alicia's medical care. We still have Alicia, and that carries no price tag.

Much can be said about local coffee shops in small towns where gossip is shared, embellished. and shared again. This happened in Tipton during Alicia's illness, as I'm sure it does in many other communities. While some just wanted a tidbit of news to share, most people truly cared and wanted to help. I was amazed at the emotional, physical and financial support we received from our small Tipton community. When we were in the hospital for weeks on end, we would come home to find that either a neighbor or a family member had mowed the lawn. Someone from our church had organized a list of church members who would bring food. Our families brought food. Our church, along with the assistance of the Aid Association for Lutherans and another local church, requested contributions to help offset some of the financial burdens we faced. Money raised by AAL and churches, along with contributions from concerned citizens, was used to replace our automatic washer. Thank goodness I didn't have to go sit at the laundromat doing laundry some night when we were home from the hospital!

COST OF CARE AND SMALL-TOWN SUPPORT

People were very generous, and I know we didn't know all the kind things that were done, nor did we ever get to thank everyone. I believe everyone who helped in any way knows how much we appreciate it, and that God watches over his earth angels. We certainly appreciate everyone's support. In the end, no matter the gossip, a small, caring community is where I want to be if ever faced with devastating news.

I referred to how we packed food from home to avoid paying for meals at the hospital. Our protocol required us to be inpatients for at least five days. Sometimes, it was just five days; sometimes, it was more. After Alicia's second surgery and once her chemotherapy was regulated, it was consistently a five-day stay. Meals for five days would have been expensive, especially since only one of us was working most of the time, allowing the other to be at the hospital with Alicia. Parking in the hospital parking ramp was another expense I found horrible. At a minimum of $7 per day, that adds up over a few days' stay. We tried not to have a car in the ramp. Generally, my parents would pick Alicia up at Grandma Timm's house and bring her to Iowa City. They would pick me up at work, and then we would go to the hospital for her next round of treatment. That way, I didn't have to pay for the car to be in the ramp. Dick could pick us up after he got off work on our last day of treatment and take us home. But we were not always so fortunate.

We spent more on parking once we reached the portion of Alicia's protocol that allowed some of the chemotherapy to be administered at home, as it was easier to have a car there on Sunday morning to take her home. I soon learned if you got up very early, took the car out of the ramp, and then put it back in, I only had to pay for the few hours between 6 a.m. and 10 a.m.

In February, Alicia received a central line, allowing her to continue her chemotherapy, tests, and treatment without having to start an IV every time. Alicia's veins were damaged by this time. Ultimately, they started IVs in her ankle or the side of her head where veins were available. She looked pretty silly with a Styrofoam cup taped to the side of her head to protect the IV site, but at least it kept her from the additional poke.

It was great (emotionally) when we could do some of her chemo in Tipton. It meant at least two fewer days in the hospital and away from the boys. The downside was the insurance company didn't want to pay for the drugs if we were at home and not hospitalized. It made absolutely no sense to me that the insurance company would rather pay $500 a day for a bed than the lesser amount to have the chemo administered at home. Apparently, they didn't think of those issues the same way we did. The insurance company also balked at paying for Alicia's central line supplies, which were several hundred dollars a month. The supplies included heparin, syringes, cleaning solution, gauze, and "windows," which were nothing more than clear skin-line pieces of covering to put over her central line to protect it and keep it clean. The insurance company would not cover the cost of these supplies, which was ridiculously high.

We made the daily flushing of Alicia's central line and changing her dressings a family affair. The boys were very curious about her central line, and I thought it was the perfect way to include them in her treatment. I was very, very nervous about her having a central line and whether I was smart enough to take care of it properly. Dr. Kisker assured me that if he didn't think I could take care of it, he would never suggest that I do so. Alicia's central line was in the center of her chest. We had to flush her central line daily (within 24 hours) and change the dressing that covered it. We would start by taking the old window dressing off and cleaning all around the site with iodine. Then, with a syringe, I would draw an exact amount of heparin from the bottle, remove the air bubbles, and then flush it into her central line to keep it open and prevent blood clotting at the opening of her line. I was so afraid of flushing an air bubble into her heart. Alicia would work her tongue like she was tasting the heparin. We were told later it was because heparin tasted salty. Then, we would finish cleaning the site and cover it with a new window to protect the line until the next day. In 24 hours, we'd start the process all over again. In the end,

COST OF CARE AND SMALL-TOWN SUPPORT

Tony could have easily changed her dressing and flushed her line all by himself. The boys were good helpers and enjoyed being a part of the entire process. Having a central line was a godsend. If, God forbid, we ever have to go back to some sort of treatment, I would highly recommend placing a central line as soon as possible.

Soon after Alicia's diagnosis, first surgery, and the start of chemotherapy, we discovered that we had a leaky roof at home. Dick's brother, Roger, offered to come and fix it. He'd take the old shingles (there were several layers) off and put new plywood and shingles on the west side of the house. That appeared to be the only real problem with the roof, and we could deal with the rest later. He had green shingles at home he would use, and he told us we could pay him whenever we could. It sounded like quite a deal, and I truly didn't care at that point what color shingles we had. They started working on the roof in August; no one could remember when it had last rained. Well, they put the sheeting on, but not well enough to withstand the strong storms we got that night. The sheeting blew up, the rain blew in, and we had a mess. Dick called me at the hospital after he got home that night and said the ceiling tiles were falling off the ceiling in Alicia's room and the wallpaper in her room, the hallway, and Tony's room was wet. I told him to close the door to Alicia's room since there wasn't anything I could do about it from the hospital, and we'd deal with it when we got home. It's interesting how what would have been a crisis on most days really didn't matter at all at that time. Eventually, we got things cleaned up and under control.

This roof episode is just another example of needing family, friends and community when faced with a devastating diagnosis. I can only imagine what families do for support when they are miles away from loved ones.

VIII
A WORLD OF UNKNOWNS

Following Alicia's cancer diagnosis, we were thrown into a world of unknowns. Again, we found ourselves standing on the outside of a window looking in at the world we were the center of. We tried to find ourselves. We were making decisions we never in our wildest dreams thought we would have to make. Certainly, the well-being of our sick child and making decisions on treatment were foremost in our minds, but the whirl around us was incredible! We still had Andy and Tony at home, so we had to figure out who would go to work and who would stay at the hospital, who went home to the other children — who needed lunch money, picture money, or field trip money — and how they were coping, and oh, yeah, someone had to keep paying the bills!

All the information we were given to consume regarding Alicia's treatment and what lay ahead, including medical terminology and prognosis, sometimes seemed insurmountable. We heard medical terms, names of tests and chemotherapy drugs that we couldn't say, spell, understand, or sometimes even remember. Still, every step of the way, we had to make decisions based on the information we were given. We were constantly learning so much we wished we never had to learn. But learn we must. We read and studied the information we received, even when the circumstances of Alicia's illness made it difficult and sometimes impossible to concentrate. A part of me just wanted to run away with Alicia or hide in a room where they couldn't find us and wish all the problems would go away. I truly wish it had been that easy.

And You Never Stop Worrying

As a parent with a child who has been sick, you will never stop worrying. As the years pass, it isn't the same gut-wrenching worry and hurt you feel at first, but not a day goes by I don't wonder about what is ahead. A child diagnosed with a life-threatening illness will never just have a stomachache, a cold, or the flu. When the boys had stomachaches, they likely ate too much or had the flu. Not with Alicia. I was always afraid it was the start of another form of cancer. I have come to believe that ignorance really is bliss. When you are hurled into this situation to begin with, you pretty much do whatever the medical professionals feel is best and suggest you do. When a child relapses or has a recurrence, you have some of the knowledge now that you didn't have the first time. Now you know too much, and still, you don't know a thing. I've always felt sorry for any parent with a medical background because they know so much more than those of us without that information. Alicia has seen too many of her friends have to go back into treatment, and some don't win their battles the second time. She knows, like we all do, it would be naïve to think the same might not or could not happen to her. She worries, but she enjoys every day she is blessed with, taking nothing for granted.

We often wonder how the treatments she received as a toddler may otherwise impact her long-term health. We already know Alicia's left hand is smaller, misshapen, and has poor circulation as a result of the dye burning her hand. And her neuroblastoma seemingly even affected her teeth. When it was time to consider braces for her teeth, she had to have eight teeth pulled before she could get her braces. These were extra teeth, some of which weren't in the right places. She had to have surgery to pull her eye teeth up into position. We are not certain the chemo played a role in the development of her teeth, especially at her young age; however, our guess is it may have. Perhaps she just had a mouthful of problems.

Alicia struggled throughout school because of learning disabilities. We know her learning disabilities were likely caused by the cancer itself and the chemotherapy she received. She has done well, however, and worked very hard to overcome many of the "labels" put on Learning Disabled (LD) kids. As an adult, Alicia has worked with adults and children with disabilities. Her cancer journey undoubtedly made her better at her job. She is currently working in a public school with middle school-aged children.

Alicia's blood pressure is the biggest problem at the moment. About the time she was 18, through routine checkups, we discovered her blood pressure was high. She had an echocardiogram, stress tests, and an ultrasound. With her history, the nephrologists were concerned there might be a tumor on her kidneys. In addition, one of the chemotherapy drugs she received was known to be hard on the patient's heart, so the doctors wanted to rule out any heart damage. The tests showed no abnormalities, and thus, her physicians assumed that either her high blood pressure was hereditary or the chemo was the cause. At 22, she had additional blood pressure problems, which doctors had difficulty regulating. Again, after some testing, they found nothing to explain why her blood pressure was out of range. This is one of those times we had to sit and wonder if the chemo might be causing her long-term problems, but it is also the time when we reminded ourselves we made the best decisions possible with the information we had.

At the age of 35, Alicia had a hysterectomy due to fibroid tumors. At 40, "soft tumors" were discovered in her abdomen and chest. Through routine MRIs and CAT scans, we are monitoring them closely in the hope there will be no growth. Little can be done regarding treatment if they start growing.

A WORLD OF UNKNOWNS

So, we have been blessed to have Alicia for an additional 40 years since she was diagnosed with neuroblastoma at not quite 2 years old. Now, although we must deal with these potential problems, we can't second-guess our original decision. But, the truth of the matter is we are never done worrying!

IX
FAMILY & FRIENDS

It is extremely important to have the love and support of family and friends when you are faced with a life-threatening diagnosis. I can't begin to explain the emotions you go through. One thing to remember is that everyone reacts differently, and there is no single pattern or right or wrong way to do so. People should think before they speak, and although there is no right or wrong way to respond to someone enduring this kind of trauma, just don't say something stupid. Those "stupid" comments are the ones we remember. Give the patient and parents a hug and let them know you are there for them.

Just as there are no real "right" ways to handle support, there are also no right and wrong ways for a family to cope with such news. Everyone has their own set of emotions and ways of coping. Please be mindful not to be critical or judgmental of people and/or families who are doing their best to cope. Unless you have been given such news, you really have no way of knowing how you would react, and it doesn't matter if you agree with someone's way of coping or not. They are doing the best they can.

One night during a hospital stay, one of the nurses came and asked me to talk to a newly diagnosed family. I didn't think I could do it, but she convinced me they needed to talk to someone who had been where they were then. We were probably six months ahead of them in our diagnosis, and the nurse thought it was important they have some support. I don't think of myself as a supportive person, and I was hesitant, but she finally convinced me to meet the family. We talked, and we cried, and we talked some more. A few weeks later, I received a nice note in the mail saying they didn't think they could have made it through those first days without me. I still don't consider myself a strong, supportive person, but apparently, all they needed was for someone to listen and understand the emotions they were going through at the time.

That brings me to why some of the strongest friendships I have are with people who were in the same shoes as we were. These people know what you are going through. It may be a different form of cancer, it may be a different-aged child, it may be "different" for any number of reasons, and still, it is the "same." I do believe moms in these circumstances grow closer to each other, perhaps for a variety of reasons, and stay closer. Perhaps it is because moms are the ones who are generally present at the hospital, maybe because they are more likely to converse with neighbors in the hall, or perhaps simply because moms feel the need to share more than dads. But, for whatever reason, I think moms grow closer to each other during these traumatic times.

We were well through chemotherapy, and I felt the need to be a part of a support group. There was no support group when we were in the midst of treatment, which always surprised me. I would have thought there might be several groups, but there weren't any. So, when a group became available, I started attending meetings. Maybe just to keep realizing how lucky we were, but I needed that. Dick never felt like he wanted to participate. We were through treatment, and he wanted to leave that part of our lives behind. Everyone handles things differently.

I'm also grateful for the friendships we have maintained with families not as fortunate as ours. It must be incredibly difficult and painful for a family that has had to deal with the loss of a child, and we still have ours.

I truly admire these people. I believe they are certainly stronger than I could be.

When Philip's family had to endure their horrific loss, it was devastating. Philip and Alicia would routinely sit in a hospital bed, IV poles with meds on either side, and they would color. Color and be children. Coloring. Something so simple in the lives of children. Each of these sessions was completed with a hug and an invitation to come do it all over again. Ladonna and I had a standing box of Kleenex that was passed between us if we weren't going to spend the entire time in the hospital together. Ladonna was there to celebrate Alicia's graduation and wedding. We stood and hugged and cried, never having to say a word to know how each other was feeling. I'll never forget the look in her eyes as I walked toward her. It had to be a bittersweet moment. They lost Philip, and we still had Alicia. I have always admired Ladonna. She is an inspiration to many. She is a truly treasured friend and has repeatedly been my rock.

I also think parents who have been in this situation better understand the important things in life. We no longer sweat the small stuff, and we've done a good job of prioritizing. Some things just don't upset us as much as they do other parents. We understand how short life is and don't plan to waste a lot of time on issues we have no control over and can do nothing about.

Just as fellow parents and support groups were important to the adults, the kids also needed support. Alicia finished her chemo and the following summer went to camp in Boone, Iowa. The camp was called Amanda the Panda Camp and was designed for children with cancer. Alicia was almost five, and I was certain she was too young to go to camp for a week, but the doctors, nurses, and camp staff convinced me to let her at least try camp. If it didn't work out, we could come get her and bring her home.

I packed her up and got her ready. I knew we would be back to get her by mid-week, that she would be homesick and wanting to come home.

Dick figured it was going to be an expensive week because I would probably want to get a motel room and stay in Boone for the week to sneak out and check on Alicia. I didn't do that! But I did know we'd be back early to get her. We got to Boone and got Alicia registered, unloaded, and to her cabin. The cabin was all decorated, and two of Alicia's counselors were her oncology nurses. I felt better immediately. Another one of her counselors was a grey-haired, grandmotherly woman whom Alicia immediately took a shine to. This same woman has been affectionately referred to for nearly 40 years as "Grandma Wilts." Grandma Wilts and her husband attended Alicia's wedding in 2004.

To say she had a marvelous time at camp is an understatement. We picked Alicia up the following Saturday afternoon, and after giving everyone hugs and packing her back in the car, Alicia cried most of the way home. She wanted to see her friends and counselors again, and she made it clear she was going back next year. That was the beginning of our camp life!

The following year, the camp underwent some administrative changes, and the name was changed to The Heart Connection Children's Cancer Programs. Oncology camp is offered one week every summer, free of charge, to any child with oncological treatment in the state of Iowa. This organization also offers a week of camp to the siblings of those oncology kids.

Alicia was a camper for the next 10 years before joining the staff as a camp counselor. She treasured seeing old friends, making new friends, and just being a regular kid. These young people go to camp looking forward to just being a "normal" kid for a week. No one spends time feeling sorry for these kids, as that would be the last thing any of them would want. They get to do activities regular kids do, and no one looks at them funny for having no hair, lost limbs, or radiation marks. Often, before the third day of camp week, many of the young male counselors have shaved their heads to resemble one or more of their campers. There is a bond between these young people. These kids all know how each other feels. There is never a need to explain. It's as if they all know what the other is thinking without saying a word.

Our boys also got involved with camp. I thought that since we were through treatment and everyone seemed to be doing fine, it would not be necessary for the boys to go to camp. The second year, they offered camp for the siblings. I let the boys go, thinking maybe they could help other siblings, or maybe they were still coping with issues that we as their parents didn't understand. That was the best thing I could have done. I don't think even the best parents can possibly understand how siblings feel or cope.

For the next 20 or so years, our kids participated in the camp as campers and then camp counselors. Eventually, Tony and his wife, Channon, were both employed by The Heart Connection Children's Cancer Programs. Dick and I, my sister Vonnie, and her late husband Harvey Dittmer volunteered as camp cooks for 10 years. We also recruited my brother, Tom, and sister, Vicki, for a number of years. Tony told me that once we were there and were a part of camp, we would always want to be a part of it. I think that's true. Every year, we fed 300 hungry staffers and campers three meals a day for eight days. This was the most rewarding thing I have ever done. And when those campers, big and small, would thank us, telling us that the meal we had prepared was the best they had ever had, it made the grueling work and long hours well worth it. Those kids appreciated everything you did for them.

The friendships made at camp are some of the strongest these kids will ever have and will last a lifetime. Losing a fellow camper is also one of the most painful things these kids endure, and believe me, they experience that loss way too often. They become family to each other, and they have connections I'm certain none of us can begin to understand. The camp staff and counselors are some of the most incredible young people I know.

FAMILY & FRIENDS

These young people need one another, through good times and bad. They instinctively know how to respond to each other's needs, wants and feelings. They have an unspoken language and understanding that binds them together. God bless them! God bless them all!!!

X
AFTER THE GOOD NEWS

We finished Alicia's chemotherapy treatments in the summer of 1985, just a little over two years from our start date. Given that her protocol was for 92 weeks, we were pleased. We experienced very few delays due to low blood counts or infections and were able to keep moving forward most of the time. Alicia had her central line for almost 18 months and, thankfully, never had an infection, which, in fact, is uncommon. Delays were frustrating because we wanted to be done with treatment. However, given the fact Alicia had surgery twice during that time, we did amazingly well. We were pleased with the timeframe in which we finished.

Post Chemo

While we were pleased when Alicia's chemo treatments ended, I will say the post-chemotherapy days were not particularly easy either. I probably did as much worrying when we finished chemo as I did during it. When we were in treatment, it seemed we had a safety net. Now we were going to stop doing what had been working. I knew we had reached the end of her protocol, and I knew her test results were good, but there was something about the security of both doing treatment and being in and out of the clinic constantly, where the health professionals were keeping a watchful eye on our little girl.

It was nice when Alicia's central line was pulled. No more flushing of her central line every 24 hours. No more supplies, needles, and medicines. No more five-day visits in the hospital . . . but also, no more security.

We were scheduled for return visits every three months. Admittedly, that doesn't sound very long. Winter is only three months away, Christmas is only three months away, and the start of school is just three months away. But when you have been in and out of the hospital every few weeks for over two years, three months is an eternity. Three months . . . 90 days . . . What could go wrong in 90 days?

Alicia seemed to feel good following the completion of her chemotherapy, and we started getting back into a normal routine at home. We went on a mini vacation to St. Louis to celebrate being done with chemo and to take the kids to Six Flags, the Zoo, and a friend's cabin in southern Missouri. The getaway trip was wonderful. Alicia couldn't get enough riding at Six Flags, and the boys had a great time.

Our first three-month checkup was in October, and of course, everyone was anxious. We all knew she was fine, but it would be so good to have this first follow-up behind us. We visited the clinic and underwent the standard blood work, chest X-rays, and other tests. Everything appeared to be fine, except her dopamine levels were high. High dopamine levels (from a 24-hour urine collection) were one of our first indications at Mercy Hospital that something was terribly wrong. My heart just sank. Because all other tests were normal, however, Dr. Kisker suggested we wait a couple of weeks and take another 24-hour collection. Perhaps something went wrong during the testing, or who knows, but we'd try it again. So, a few weeks later, we did another 24-hour collection and went in for some additional scans and tests to see if something was going on again in her little body. The X-rays and scans were clear, but again, the dopamine levels were elevated. Dr. Kisker told us he could find no apparent reason for her levels to be so elevated. Since we had not had a reading of her dopamine levels before her cancer, he said, maybe she just had abnormally high levels, and what we were seeing now was really her normal. He suggested making an appointment at either a research hospital in L.A. (where her original biopsy was sent), Mayo Clinic in Rochester, Minnesota, where they were doing major research with neuroblastoma, or wait a few weeks and try running the dopamine tests again. Waiting a few weeks was really not an option for me. I wanted to know something NOW. Since Rochester was more easily accessible, both geographically and financially, we opted for Mayo and asked him to make the appointments.

As soon as our appointments at Mayo were scheduled, we contacted the Cedar County Health Care office to see if they could assist us in making affordable housing arrangements in Rochester. God bless Rosie. This woman was incredible and made phone calls and arrangements for us without missing a beat. She found an upstairs apartment we could rent for however long we needed and at a minimal rate. It was a two-bedroom apartment with a small kitchen and bathroom, located just about a block from the entrance to Mayo, where we could walk the rest of the way underground and through a warm tunnel.

The apartment itself was very old and not very warm, but we managed just fine. It was so nice to have a kitchen so we could fix some of our meals rather than going to restaurants. Not only was this easier financially, but it was also nice not to have to go out in the cold again at night. Rosie had indicated we would have kitchen facilities, so I had packed accordingly. We took some groceries and essentials, so we could stay with Alicia as much as possible. It was so cold when we arrived in Rochester that when we opened the trunk lid to start unpacking, the coffee carafe exploded. We had shattered glass everywhere and nothing to make coffee in. Oh, well, life was going to go on.

AFTER THE GOOD NEWS

Knowing the boys were again going to be left behind, Rosie had packed a box of groceries with "special things" for them to have at Grandma's. There were some canned goods to help Grandma with some of the meals. There were some fun snack foods they normally didn't have at home, and an activity book for each of them. One was a punch-out, put-together, cowboy/rodeo scene, and I don't remember the other one. But the very best of all, at least according to the boys, was a box of Captain Crunch WITH crunch berries. That was a real treat for them and certainly the best part of the entire box. Rosie knew just how to make this trip easier for everyone!

The Sunday before Thanksgiving 1985, we packed our boys off to Grandma's house. We had some hugs and tears. With Alicia in the car, we headed north to Rochester, Minnesota. I remember it being a bright, sunshiny, cold day. I also remember having this horrible lump in the pit of my stomach. I just didn't want to start all over. I just couldn't imagine our little girl being sick again and all the what-ifs. I didn't want to do this, but still, I knew I couldn't just sit and wait. Doing nothing was not an option.

When we arrived in Rochester and unpacked, I went downstairs to use the public phone (no cell phones back then) to call home and let everyone know we had arrived safely. I talked to Grandma Timm and the boys, and although they wanted us to be home again, they seemed to be doing fine. Then I called my folks, and I don't know why, but I just lost it. I started to cry and couldn't seem to get it back together. I think the reality of being back in the throes of this mess was finally coming down around me. I'd made it through packing again, leaving the boys behind and arriving in Rochester, but now I felt like the world was closing in. After talking to the folks and having a good cry, I went back upstairs to Dick and Alicia to fix some supper and get settled in for the night. We were to be at the clinic early, before 7 a.m., so I wanted to get Alicia through her bath and to bed fairly early.

Monday morning, we arrived at our designated spot for registration. We were the only ones in a huge room lined with what appeared to be hundreds of bright-colored chairs. Apparently, the color of the chairs had something to do with the organization of all those people and particular clinics or labs. We got registered and sat in the brightly colored chairs for only a matter of minutes when someone came to get us and take us to the testing area. It seemed in no time at all, we were getting ready for Alicia's scans, and everything was underway. She had to drink a large amount of solution before her scan, but as soon as she'd done that, we were ready to roll. Since I could stay right at her side, we decided to try doing the scan (about two hours in length) without sedation. She had to lie perfectly still, but I could be there and hold her hand and talk to her the entire time. She did amazingly well. At one point, she even fell asleep for a little while. When they completed her scan, we were free to go for the day. We wandered around in the tunnels of the Mayo Clinic for some time, just to see how incredibly huge their institution was and to kill time. We eventually returned to the apartment to rest for a bit. Then we got in the car and went for a little ride to see some of Rochester. We saw the Canadian geese on the lake and marveled at how many hundreds of them there were.

We stopped at a little grocery store so Dick could pick up pickled pigs' feet for supper. Little did he know he was going to have to share with his daughter. I'll never forget those two sitting in front of the TV watching Ewoks and eating pickled pigs' feet, onions, bread, and butter. Alicia was perfectly content and to this day, she talks about staying in her "little house" at the "big hospital," watching Ewoks, and eating pickled pigs' feet with her Daddy. While they were so engaged, I decided to take a long, hot bath in an old claw-footed tub, which I found very inviting.

Mid-morning on Tuesday, we were due back at Mayo. Again, we didn't have to sit and wait for anyone. Everything went incredibly smoothly. Although I never asked, it seemed that since we were part of this research project, we didn't have to wait anywhere for anyone. We met with the doctor conducting the research study. He told us there was nothing suspicious on any of the scans. While this was wonderful news, it still didn't answer the question of why Alicia's dopamine level was so high. He suggested that since nothing was detected on the scans done on Monday, we did not need to subject Alicia to any further testing. Rather, he suggested we go home, try to be patient, and do the 24-hour urine collection again when Dr. Kisker thought it was necessary. It was beginning to look more and more like Alicia's levels were just going to run high.

Oh . . . that word "patience."

We decided to go back to the apartment and pack our belongings. Although it was going to be a long day and we'd be getting home late, we wanted to get home and see the boys. We made it before they were in bed, so we got to take them home with us. It was so good to be back home. Although we had been hosting Thanksgiving for several years, we decided we would not be able to do so this year. Mom had us come to Durant to eat BBQ ribs on Thanksgiving. Hardly traditional, but it was so good, and even more wonderful to be home with no new serious health issues. I believe my family has been generally thankful every day since our original diagnosis, but Thanksgiving seemed particularly special.

We began by monitoring Alicia's dopamine levels and testing them regularly. Her levels continued to be high, and other tests were always good, so we stopped worrying somewhat about the dopamine levels. We resumed our schedule of checkups every three months and remained on that schedule for two years. Then we went to six-month checks and then to annual checks.

I was stressed with every appointment and anxious every time they extended the length between visits.

So, when Dr. Kisker said, "OK, we'll see you in two years."

I replied, "TWO YEARS?"

When he said, "Yes, two years."

I said, "No, I can't wait two years. I can't sit and wonder if something has been going on in her body for two years!"

Dr. Kisker looked at me and said, "Peggy, you are a good mom. You will know if something isn't right, and you will bring her in. In the meantime, if you are just going through withdrawal, come on in and sit in the lobby or the clinic waiting room until you feel better, but there really is no reason for us to see her any sooner than that."

OH, easy for him to say!

I was determined I couldn't wait two years between visits. But you know what? Those two years went flying by, and all of a sudden, it was time to return for a check-up. Of course, I had to stew myself into a frenzy by the time appointment day arrived. At one of our checkup appointments, we were sitting, waiting to have blood work done, when a family was told their child had relapsed. I was instantly sick to my stomach and felt like I just needed to run and get some air. Since I couldn't leave Alicia, I had no choice but to regroup, suck it up, and stay put. Although every family is perfectly clear those could easily be words they will hear again, the sound of those words will ALWAYS be a nightmare. I can't imagine how you pick up and start all over again.

One fall Sunday morning, probably six or seven years later, when I was out working in the yard and raking up leaves, Alicia came out to tell me she felt a lump in her breast. Trying not to panic, I told her I would be in in a few minutes to look at it and see what she was talking about. Again, I was instantly sick to my stomach. I was angry, I was scared, and I was crying. The madder I got, the faster I raked, and the more tears fell, the colder I got, so I kept raking and raking and raking. Hoping, I guess, that by the time I got into the house, nothing was really going to be wrong.

Yes, there was something we could feel in her right breast. It didn't hurt her, but there was something there. On Monday morning, I called the clinic, and of course, they thought she should be seen as soon as possible. The oncology clinic would write orders for Alicia to have a mammogram. Here is my pre-teen girl to whom I now have to explain this whole procedure. I promised I would be with her as much as they would let me and we would get through this, too. Following her mammogram, the doctor came in almost immediately. Yes, there was something there, but he was inclined to believe it was likely scar tissue and wanted to keep a close eye on it. He thought if there was no change in the immediate future, that was probably what it was, and we shouldn't be concerned. I remember hugging her so tight she said, "MOM, I CAN'T BREATHE!" "Tough, I NEED to hug you!" I felt such a profound sense of relief. Today, the spot is still there and hasn't changed. Another sigh of relief.

Over the next several years, there were more visits and check-ups, more check-ups and visits. . . It seemed like a never-ending cycle, but one we knew we had to stick with. With a history like Alicia's, you just don't take any chances by missing appointments or tests. You have to constantly stay on top of everything.

In the fall of her junior year in high school, during a routine check-up, we discovered that Alicia's blood pressure was elevated. This was a surprise. Something we hadn't had before. We had seen low iron, and she seemed to require more sleep than most young people her age, but we always assumed that was a side effect of the chemotherapy. Well, what to do now with elevated blood pressure? Oh, let the testing begin. There was, of course, concern there may be a tumor somewhere again, elevating her blood pressure. She may be having kidney trouble. There may be a tumor on her kidneys. The oncology clinic immediately arranged with the nephrology clinic for Alicia to meet with doctors there and schedule an ultrasound to determine if there was a tumor on her kidneys. So, Dick, Alicia and I were off to ultrasound for this test. I think Dick knew how stressed I was and thought it was best if he was there too. It didn't take very long for them to call Alicia's name, and Dick decided he was just going to wander the clinic halls a little while. An elderly couple was sitting at one end of the waiting room, and I was alone at the other end. Soon after Alicia left for her test, a mom pushed a boy, he appeared 10-12 years old, into the waiting room in his wheelchair. He had two IV poles, not a hair on his head, and a mask over his face to protect him from infections. I immediately felt like I couldn't breathe. It all looked too familiar, and I just couldn't come to grips with the thought of Alicia being sick again. The mom parked the boy close to me and then left the room. Soon, a nurse came and took him to another room. Whew. I just sat and took deep breaths, trying to block the image of him sitting in that chair. Another young life interrupted by this damn disease. Another kid who had to give so much of his childhood. No one ever said life was fair . . . cancer is a constant reminder of that.

The ultrasound didn't take long, and afterwards we were directed back to the renal clinic. After meeting with the renal doctor again, he said it would likely be the next day before they had any answers. He also said it was unlikely there was a tumor, and it was not neuroblastoma, but another form of cancer might be causing her problems. They could no doubt tell I was a basket case and promised to call on Friday as soon as they had results. The nurse who was involved in our visit was exceptional. She was comforting and was the one who agreed to let us know as soon as they knew something. Thursday, about 8 p.m., she called the house. She had gotten results and didn't want us to worry all night. The ultrasound was clear. No signs of tumor. So, we didn't have an answer to the high blood pressure issue, but we didn't have a tumor, at least on her kidneys, to fight. We were all so relieved to hear that news, we didn't think to ask what was next. I so appreciated the call. That same nurse proved to be a wonderful person time and time again.

Friday morning, I called the renal clinic and thanked them again for letting us know so quickly. I also needed to find out how we were to proceed and what, if any, tests they would conduct. The following Tuesday, we were advised that Alicia should have a stress test and a couple more scans. Those were all quickly scheduled, and, again, everything looked OK. They were starting to believe her history and family history of high blood pressure may be the cause of her elevated readings, although she really was too young for such issues. A few days later, I got a call to bring Alicia to the pediatric cardiology clinic. Someone who had read the scans and stress test results wasn't as convinced there was nothing there. Since one of her chemotherapy drugs was known to be hard on hearts, it made sense there may have been something showing now that may be causing problems. During chemo, no heart damage had been detected, but after several years, that possibility existed. Of course, we couldn't get in until the next week, and the day happened to be Dick's birthday. We all went together again and met with two pediatric cardiologists who felt her scans and her stress test results were normal. They weren't sure what the technician might have seen, but they were comfortable, agreeing there was nothing suspicious. What a huge relief.

So, back to the renal clinic, where we would get Alicia started on some medication. It would likely take some time to regulate her blood pressure. They would start her on a very low dose and increase the dosage and/or types of medications until the right combination was found. Although I hate the fact she will be on high blood pressure medicine for the rest of her life, not finding tumors anywhere was a relief. My hospital friend Ladonna said we'd NEVER be done worrying. She's absolutely right.

Alicia spent time at the renal clinic and in the doctors' offices, ensuring her blood pressure was regulated and that she received the right combination of medications. She visited the renal clinic that June and received a good report regarding her blood pressure readings. It seemed everything was working out, and she just needed to take care of herself, monitor her diet, and, of course, get some exercise. They wanted to see her back in about six months.

In July, less than one month later, while we were working and Alicia and the boys were attending the Amanda Panda camp, one of the camp nurses came to the kitchen to tell me that Alicia's blood pressure was extremely high and they had sent someone to pick up special medicine to help lower it. KIDS!!! We never figured out that episode, but we returned to the renal clinic as soon as possible after coming home from camp. Her blood pressure was fine, and it appeared her meds were working. People wonder why I look so old!

FINISHING UP MY THOUGHTS...

Nearly 40 years ago I had the idea of putting some of my thoughts about our storm on paper hoping to benefit new families in the pediatric clinic. Finishing those thoughts has taken longer than I imagined, and it's turned into a larger project. We've been out of treatment for a long time now, and although there have been some pretty big bumps in the road, we still have Alicia. There is no doubt, over the past 40-plus years, many things have changed regarding treatment, research, and education of neuroblastoma and all forms of children's cancer.

In 2008, Alicia's heart doctor in the Quad-Cities referred her to the UIHC, saying she was likely going to need a heart transplant. I immediately contacted my former boss Dr. David Skorton, who, in addition to serving as the Vice President for Research at The University of Iowa, where I supported him, was also a pediatric cardiologist. Since Alicia was an adult, he referred us to Dr. Richard Kerber. After meeting with the doctors at UIHC, additional testing, and some changes in her medicines, she has been able to postpone a transplant. I tell her every day she can hold on to her heart; someone is coming up with a medical miracle.

More than 40 years is a long time. Tony and Andy are happily married men with children. Dick is a cancer survivor. Alicia has become a grandma. I've become a great grandma. Many life decisions have been made, some better than others . . .

But life goes on . . .

We are eternally grateful to the UIHC and its professionals for helping us through this medical journey. Doctors, nurses, therapists, unit clerks, technicians, secretaries, housekeeping staff —everyone we encountered every day, thank you. To all the families we met and to those who became friends through a disease no one should have to face, we are thankful. To our family, friends, and the Tipton community, who supported us, we couldn't have survived this without you.

My initial intention in putting some thoughts into writing was just to help newly diagnosed families know they were not alone. There are no words to explain the emotions that come with receiving a life-threatening diagnosis. Just remember, you're not the first ones, you're not the last. You are not alone.

-Peggy

ACKNOWLEDGMENT

My heartfelt thanks to Stephana Colbert for her encouragement, faith, and support of me in completing this book. My initial purpose was hoping to help newly diagnosed families know they weren't alone when hearing their child has cancer. Stephana helped me see there is still a need for this project.